CERVAGEM
gemeprost

A new prostaglandin in obstetrics and gynaecology

Acknowledgement

The Editor wishes to thank Mr A. J. Christmas of May & Baker Ltd. for his valuable assistance with the editing of this book.

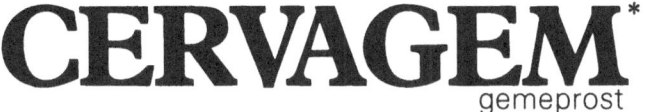

CERVAGEM*
gemeprost

A new prostaglandin in obstetrics and gynaecology

Edited by Sultan M. M. Karim

Proceedings of a Symposium held at the Shangri-La Hotel, Singapore, 31 July 1982.
Organised by May & Baker Ltd, Essex, England

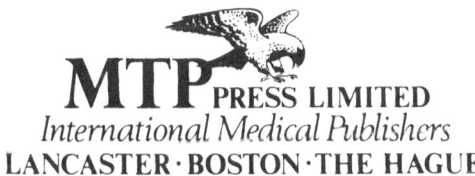

MTP **PRESS LIMITED**
International Medical Publishers
LANCASTER · BOSTON · THE HAGUE

*CERVAGEM is a trade mark for products containing gemeprost (I.N.N.) developed by
May & Baker Ltd., and the Rhône-Poulenc Group

Published in the
United Kingdom and Europe by
MTP Press Limited
Falcon House
Lancaster, England

British Library Cataloguing in Publication Data

Cervagem: a new prostaglandin in obstetrics and gynaecology.

1. Human reproduction—Congresses
2. Cervagem—Congresses
I. Karim, Sultan M. M.   II. May & Baker Limited
612'.6   QP251
ISBN-13: 978-94-011-7300-1   e-ISBN-13: 978-94-011-7298-1
DOI: 10.1007/978-94-011-7298-1

Published in the USA by
MTP Press
A division of Kluwer Boston Inc.
190 Old Derby Street
Hingham, MA 02043, USA

Library of Congress Cataloging in Publication Data

Main entry under title:

Cervagem: a new prostaglandin in obstetrics and gynaecology.

Bibliography: p.
Includes index.
1. Prostaglandins—Physiological effect—Congresses.
2. Uterus, Pregnant—Effect of drugs on—Congresses.
3. Generative organs, Female—Effect of drugs on—Congresses.
4. Obstetrical pharmacology—Congresses.
I. Karim, Sultan M. M.   [DNLM: 1. Prostaglandins E,
Synthetic—Congresses. 2. Dilatation—Methods—Congresses.
3. Abortifacient agents—Congresses. QV 175 C419 1982]
RG129.P7C47 1982   618   83–706

ISBN-13: 978-94-011-7300-1

Phototypeset by Blackpool Typesetting Services Ltd., Blackpool

Butler & Tanner Limited, Frome and London

Contents

List of speakers

Mr Tan Joo Hock
Pharmaceutical Manager
May & Baker Ltd
(Singapore Branch)
14 Chin Bee Road
Jurong, Singapore 2261

Dr James A. McFadzean
Director of Research
May & Baker Ltd
Dagenham, Essex RM10 7XS,
England

Dr Keith Crowshaw
Prostaglandin Products Coordinator
May & Baker Ltd
Dagenham, Essex RM10 7XS,
England

Dr Sultan M. M. Karim
(Symposium Chairman and
Proceedings Editor)
Research Professor of Obstetrics
and Gynaecology
Department of Obstetrics
and Gynaecology
National University of Singapore
Kandang Kerbau Hospital
Hampshire Road, Singapore 0821

Dr Pak Chung Ho
Lecturer
Department of Obstetrics
and Gynaecology
Queen Mary Hospital
University of Hong Kong
Pokfulam Road, Hong Kong

Dr Petter R. Fylling
Associate Professor and
Head of Department of
Obstetrics and Gynaecology
Ullevol Hospital
Oslo, Norway

Mrs Susan A. Pitts
Clinical Research Department
May & Baker Ltd
Dagenham, Essex RM10 7XS,
England

Dr Marc Bygdeman
Professor
Department of Women's Diseases
Karolinska Hospital
S-104 01 Stockholm, Sweden

Dr K. Satoh
Associate Professor
Department of Obstetrics
and Gynaecology
University of Tokyo
School of Medicine
7-3-1 Bunkyo-Ku, Tokyo, Japan

Dr Allan Salem
International Medical Development
Manager
May & Baker Ltd
Dagenham, Essex RM10 7XS,
England

INVITED CONTRIBUTOR

Dr M. G. Elder
Professor of Obstetrics
and Gynaecology
Institute of Obstetrics
and Gynaecology
Hammersmith Hospital
London, England

Introduction

Honourable Chairman, distinguished speakers, ladies and gentlemen, May & Baker, Singapore is proud to play a part in organizing and hosting this symposium. I hope that it is not necessary for me to introduce myself, as Singapore doctors have received my letter of invitation and overseas delegates have received my letter of welcome. It is my very pleasant duty to introduce our Director of Research, Dr J. A. McFadzean, who has come specially to grace this occasion.

Dr McFadzean, Sir, may I invite you to say a few words to this gathering of distinguished participants.

Tan Joo Hock

Welcome

It is my privilege on behalf of May & Baker to welcome you here today.

We have representatives from nine countries – Singapore, Malaysia, Thailand, Hong Kong, Indonesia, Japan, Norway, Sweden and UK.

It is appropriate that this Symposium on Cervagem be held in South-east Asia where so much excellent development work was done with this product.

Cervagem has resulted from many years of collaborative research and development between May & Baker and the Ono Pharmaceutical Company of Japan. It has been a most happy collaboration from the time the active ingredient ONO-802 was synthesized by the Ono Company.

You will hear today of the stage we have reached with the R & D work.

I wish you a most fruitful Symposium and I now have the privilege of introducing to you your Chairman, Professor Sultan Karim. When one thinks of prostaglandins in the field of obstetrics, one thinks of Sultan Karim as the father, if not the grandfather.

Professor Karim, I have much pleasure in asking you to take the chair.

J. A. McFadzean

Chairman's opening remarks

Thank you, Dr McFadzean, for your generous introduction, and for your invitation to chair this afternoon's proceedings. I believe most of you as practising obstetricians and gynaecologists have some experience in the use of prostaglandins in your discipline. As a result of their widespread use, the limitations of first generation prostaglandins (particularly in terms of side-effects) are now recognized. Attempts to improve their utility come through development of new analogues and Cervagem is the latest addition to a list of such compounds whose potential in obstetrics and gynaecology is being explored. Amongst the speakers, we have people with many years of experience in developing the practical application of prostaglandins, including Cervagem. We also have experts from the WHO Prostaglandin Task Force Steering Committee which has for many years been involved in organizing multicentre clinical trials in many countries. With their expertise and the experience of many in the audience we should have an exciting afternoon's discussion.

I am impressed with the attendance this afternoon which could only reflect the interest prostaglandins have generated amongst obstetricians and gynaecologists. To get the proceedings going, may I invite Dr Keith Crowshaw from May & Baker, who has been involved in the development of Cervagem from the very beginning, to give us a talk on the basic pharmacology of Cervagem.

Sultan M. M. Karim
Singapore 1982

1
Comparison of the pharmacological and biochemical properties of ONO-802 (Cervagem) and the naturally occurring prostaglandins

K. CROWSHAW

INTRODUCTION

A range of very potent biologically active compounds are biosynthesized from the 20-carbon polyunsaturated fatty acids in mammalian species. Arachidonic acid is the most abundant of these fatty acids and there are known to be two major pathways of interest (Figure 1.1). The first, involving specific lipoxygenase action on arachidonic acid, leads to the formation of hydroxy-acids, leukotrienes and slow-reacting substance of anaphylaxis. The other pathway, which was first described nearly 20 years ago, involves the initial formation of the very unstable, very potent cyclo-endoperoxides PGG_2 and PGH_2. From these intermediates different enzymes can form prostacyclins on the one hand, and thromboxanes on the other.

The compounds I shall discuss in some detail are prostaglandin E_2 (PGE_2) and prostaglandin $F_{2\alpha}$ ($PGF_{2\alpha}$), which are also formed from the cyclo-endoperoxides. The chemical structures of these two prostaglandins (Table 1.1) differ only in one respect; $PGF_{2\alpha}$ has an alcohol function in place of the 9-ketone function in PGE_2. This small difference leads to profound differences in biological potency. Two items of similarity are that both compounds have weak or negligible effects on platelets, and they both are very potent in contracting smooth muscle,

1

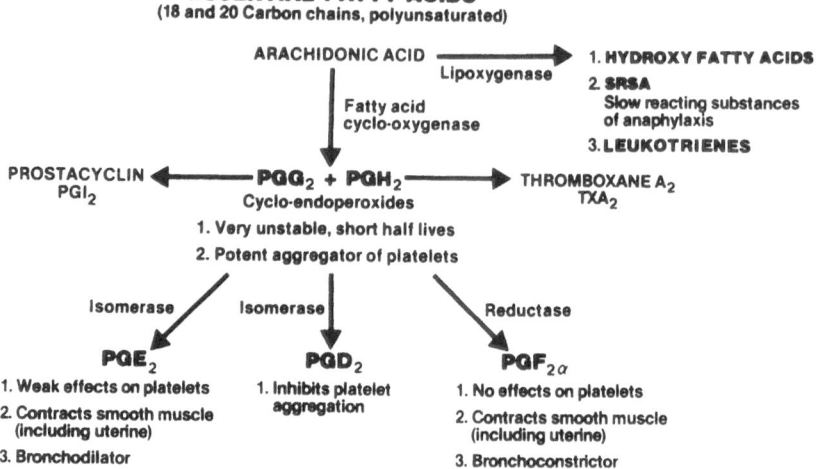

Figure 1.1   The arachidonic acid cascade

including uterine smooth muscle. The difference appears in the bronchodilator activity of the compounds. PGE_2 is a very potent bronchodilator and it is also a very strong vasodilator. $PGF_{2\alpha}$, on the other hand, is a potent bronchoconstrictor and is also a vasoconstrictor[1,2].

Table 1.1   Structure and pharmacological actions of PGE_2 and $PGF_{2\alpha}$

Structure	Activity on smooth muscle (non-vascular)	Blood pressure	Renal blood flow	Sodium excretion	Removal by lung
$PGF_{2\alpha}$	Contract	↓	↑	↑	Yes
PGE_2	Contract	↑	?	?	Yes

PROSTAGLANDINS AND REPRODUCTION

These two prostaglandins, PGE_2 and $PGF_{2\alpha}$, were first isolated from ram seminal vesicles and, soon afterwards, Samuelsson's group[3,4] in Sweden isolated large concentrations from human seminal plasma. These initial associations of PGE_2 and $PGF_{2\alpha}$ with the male reproductive system were soon overshadowed by evidence suggesting that these prostaglandins had important functions as hormones involved in female reproductive processes.

In Chapter 2, Professor Karim will describe in more detail the clinical applications of PGE_2 and $PGF_{2\alpha}$ and I shall simply present the background here (see Table 1.2). The first demonstration that prostaglandins were associated with female reproduction was by Professor Pickles in the United Kingdom; he showed[5] that menstrual fluid contains appreciable concentrations of PGE_2 and $PGF_{2\alpha}$. Soon afterwards Professor Bygdeman, who worked on isolated strips of human uterine tissue, showed that these two prostaglandins can contract and/or relax uterine strips obtained from patients at various stages of the cycle and pregnancy[6]. This was followed by the work of Professor Karim, who found that amniotic fluid[7] and placental cord of women[8] contains large concentrations of $PGF_{2\alpha}$. He subsequently went on to show that $PGF_{2\alpha}$ is present in the peripheral blood of women in labour but, interestingly, not in large concentrations in the blood before labour[9]. Finally, in animal studies, both PGE_2 and $PGF_{2\alpha}$ have been shown to stimulate contractions of uterine smooth muscle *in vivo* (references in Kirton[10]).

Table 1.2 Prostaglandins and reproduction

1. HUMAN SEMINAL PLASMA (Samuelsson *et al.*)[3,4]	Contains large concentrations of PGE_2, $PGF_{2\alpha}$ and 19-OH PGs
2. MENSTRUAL FLUID (Pickles *et al.*)[5]	Contains PGE_2 and $PGF_{2\alpha}$
3. HUMAN UTERINE TISSUE (Bygdeman)[6]	Isolated strips contract and/or relax to PGE_2 and $PGF_{2\alpha}$
4. HUMAN PLACENTAL CORD (Karim)[8]	Contains $PGF_{2\alpha}$
5. LABOUR (Karim)[9]	$PGF_{2\alpha}$ is present in amniotic fluid, decidua and peripheral blood of women in labour (but not before)
6. ANIMAL STUDIES[10]	PGE_2 and $PGF_{2\alpha}$ stimulate contractions of uterine smooth muscle

Table 1.3   Induction of labour by PGE_2 and $PGF_{2\alpha}$

Clinical studies:	PGE_2 and $PGF_{2\alpha}$ are effective agents for induction of labour
Administration:	Intravenous, extra-amniotic Vaginal Oral(PGE_2)
Side-effects:	Nausea Vomiting Diarrhoea Dysmenorrhoeic pain Fever Headache
Additional benefit:	Ripening of the cervix

These observations obviously led obstetricians, gynaecologists and researchers to suggest that the prostaglandins might well be useful pharmacological agents to induce labour at term, and this, in fact, was demonstrated. Clinical studies have shown that both PGE_2 and $PGF_{2\alpha}$ are effective agents for the induction of labour (Table 1.3). Various routes of administration have been used, including intravenous, extra-amniotic and vaginal. In the case of PGE_2 there are oral tablets available which are effective for induction of labour at term. The side-effects observed are what we now know to be the typical side-effects of prostaglandins, the commonest being nausea, vomiting and diarrhoea. Less commonly observed side-effects are dysmenorrhoeic pain, fever and headache. An additional benefit arising from the use of PGE_2 and to some extent $PGF_{2\alpha}$ for this indication is ripening of the cervix. The use of these two prostaglandins for induction of labour has been well reviewed by Karim[11].

Following this work investigators then thought that the prostaglandins might induce second trimester abortion and, indeed, they are effective (Table 1.4). Several routes of administration (intravenous,

Table 1.4   Prostaglandins and second trimester abortion

Administration:	Intravenous Intra-amniotic Extra-amniotic Vaginal
Side-effects:	Comparable to induction of labour ↑↑ Vaginal pessaries (20 mg PGE_2) (Reports of uterine rupture)
Additional benefit:	Cervical dilatation

intra-amniotic, extra-amniotic and vaginal) have been used. Side-effects are comparable to those seen in labour induction, but may be more severe since the dosage required to induce abortion is quite high for some of the routes of administration. There is a vaginal pessary formulation containing 20 mg of PGE_2 which can cause a high incidence of side-effects including reports of uterine rupture[12]. The use of prostaglandins for therapeutic second trimester abortions is preferable to earlier methods of inducing abortion, such as hypertonic saline and urea/saline. Moreover, there is the additional benefit in that the cervix is dilated by the prostaglandins, which is an aid to the abortion procedure.

Both PGE_2 and $PGF_{2\alpha}$ have been commercially available for a number of years. The Upjohn Company and the Ono Pharmaceutical Company both supply these products for induction of labour and for second trimester termination of pregnancy. There are, however, major factors which limit the usefulness of the natural prostaglandins as abortifacients. The first of these is their chemical instability. The prostaglandins (PGE_2 specifically) under the influence of water, air and heat, can lose the elements of water chemically from the molelcule (Figure 1.2). The beta-ketone structure is unstable and breaks down leading to the formation of PGA_2 and subsequently to PGB_2, both of which are relatively inactive pharmacologically. However, pharmaceutical chemists and formulation experts can now formulate PGE_2 in ways which overcome this difficulty to some extent, and most products available have shelf lives of up to 2 years when stored at 4 °c.

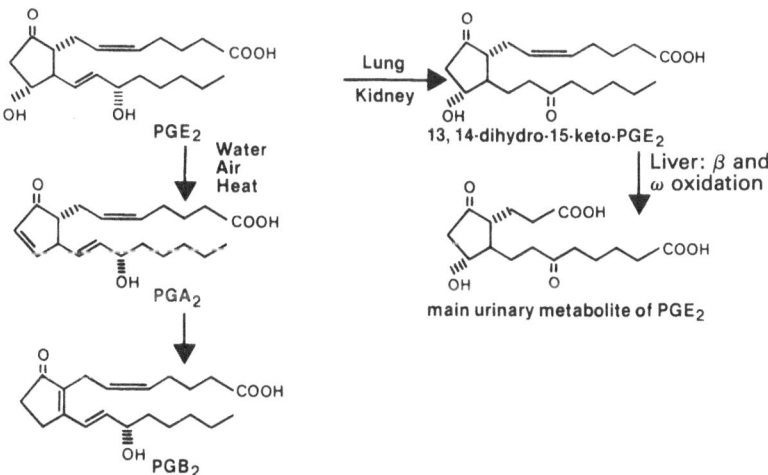

Figure 1.2 Stability and metabolism of the natural prostaglandins

5

A much more serious limitation is the metabolic instability of PGE_2 and of $PGF_{2\alpha}$. Figure 1.2 illustrates the metabolism of PGE_2. There are enzymes in the lung and in the kidney which are able to transform PGE_2 to the relatively inactive metabolite 13,14-dihydro-15-keto PGE_2. To give an example of the activity of this enzyme – once PGE_2 is absorbed into the blood stream, one passage across the lung will transform over 95% of the PGE_2 to this metabolite[13]. Further metabolism in the liver by both β- and ω-oxidation leads to the formation of a dicarboxylic acid, which has lost four carbons, and this is the main urinary metabolite of PGE_2. All the known metabolites of PGE_2 are very much less potent pharmacologically and biologically than the parent compound.

Numerous attempts have been made to use PGE_2 and $PGF_{2\alpha}$ for first trimester abortion[14]. However, even after extra-ovular administration, the results have not been very good and quite high doses are required. It is for this reason that considerable effort has been devoted by pharmaceutical chemists to the synthesis of more potent, metabolically stable analogues. A major part of this effort has been devoted to preparing luteolytic prostaglandins and I would now like briefly to discuss luteolysis.

Luteolysis

In animals, the importance of progesterone production by the corpus luteum during the luteal phase of the menstrual cycle and during early pregnancy is well established. Any procedure which results in the premature regression of the corpus luteum with an associated decrease in progesterone production is called luteolysis. In subprimates, primarily laboratory animals and farm animals, $PGF_{2\alpha}$ is effective in causing luteolysis, both in the pregnant and non-pregnant cycle. PGE_2 is approximately ten times less potent as a luteolytic in these species[11]. This property has been utilized in the development of $PGF_{2\alpha}$ and its analogues (Figure 1.3) for oestrus synchronization in farm animals[15].

It was hoped that these or similar analogues of $PGF_{2\alpha}$ could be developed as luteolytic agents to induce early abortion in women. The rationale for this is that, in women, maintenance of pregnancy up to the seventh week depends on progesterone production by a functional corpus luteum. A luteolytic prostaglandin, if active in women, would be expected to cause regression of the corpus luteum and cessation of progesterone production, leading to interruption of the pregnancy and induction of menstruation. However, to date, none

6

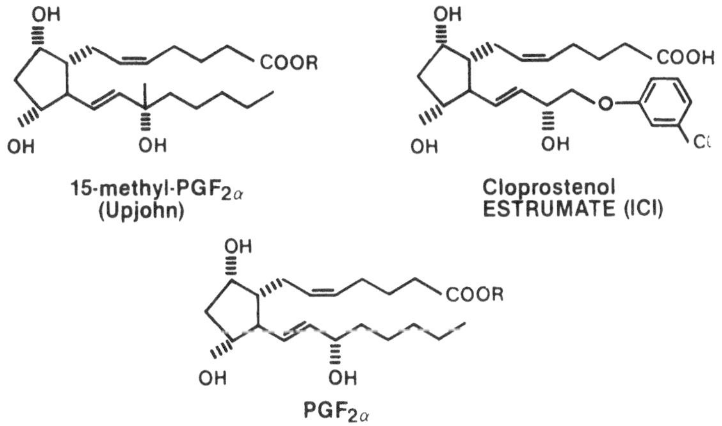

Figure 1.3 Structures of prostaglandin $F_{2\alpha}$ analogues clinically tested as luteolytics

of the prostaglandins or their analogues has been clearly demonstrated to be luteolytic in women or primates[11]. Even the ICI series of 16-phenoxy $PGF_{2\alpha}$ analogues, including Estrumate, which are some of the most potent luteolytic agents produced, have been reported to be relatively ineffective as early abortifacients in women[16].

Uterine stimulants: ONO-802 (Cervagem)

In 1974, in collaboration with the Ono Pharmaceutical Company, we at May & Barker decided that the available evidence at that time justified a search for analogues of PGE_1 and PGE_2 with potent uterine stimulant properties in an effort to find an effective agent for very early abortion. We were also concerned that such an agent should be a potent cervical dilator. There are, however, many points to be considered when planning the synthesis of prostaglandin analogues. Such analogues should have chemical stability and be as resistant as possible to biochemical inactivation. Chemists have a number of ways of doing this. I have mentioned that the lung contains very active enzymes which metabolize PGE_2 and $PGF_{2\alpha}$ to inactive metabolites. By placing methyl groups at the 15- and/or 16-position of the prostaglandin molecule, rapid metabolism by these enzymes can be prevented. Analogues of this type have been made, and are in fact very much more potent than their parent prostaglandins. They are, however, still susceptible to other routes of metabolism such as β- and ω-oxidation.

After reviewing the screening data on over 1,000 prostaglandin analogues, ONO-802 (gemeprost) was selected as being a suitable

7

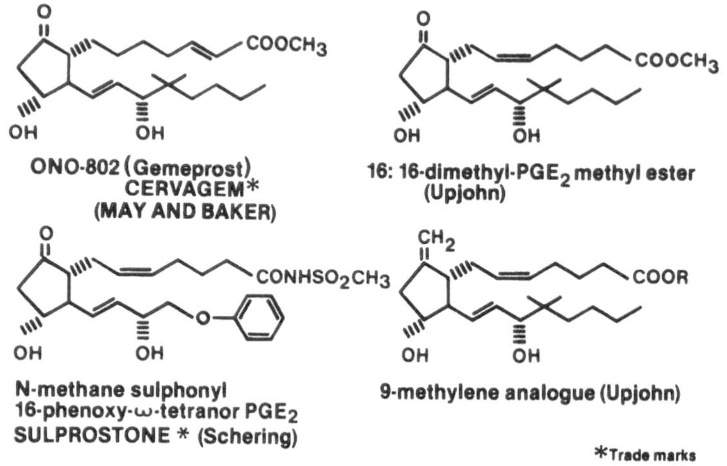

Figure 1.4   Structures of prostaglandin E analogues undergoing clinical evaluation

candidate for clinical evaluation (Figure 1.4). This compound is a potent uterine stimulant with greatly increased selectivity of action with regard to side-effects when compared to both PGE_2 and $PGF_{2\alpha}$. The 16,16-dimethyl group confers increased metabolic stability, for the reasons mentioned above. Gemeprost is the approved name of the compound and Cervagem is the May & Baker trade name. However, most previous publications refer to the compound by its research number, ONO-802, and all three names may be used at times during this symposium. Three other prostaglandin E analogues from other companies are also currently undergoing clinical evaluation (Figure 1.4). Sulprostone (Schering)[17] parallels ICI's Estrumate[16] (Figure 1.3) in utilizing a 16-phenoxy group, which also hinders metabolism of the compound by the route described above. However, Sulprostone appears to be relatively ineffective by the vaginal route[17], its recommended route of administration being intramuscular. The Upjohn compound 16,16-dimethyl PGE_2 methyl ester, being a PGE_2 analogue, is chemically less stable than the corresponding PGE_1 analogues and Upjohn scientists have been devoting their attention to the novel 9-methylene analogue (Figure 1.4). Replacement of the 9-ketone group of PGE_2 with a 9-methylene group leads to a chemically stable product but it is much less potent than the analogue from which it was derived [18, 19]. It is also about 35–70 times less potent than gemeprost as a uterine stimulant, based on the clinical doses used to induce abortion (1 mg for ONO-802, 35 or 70 mg for the 9-methylene analogue).

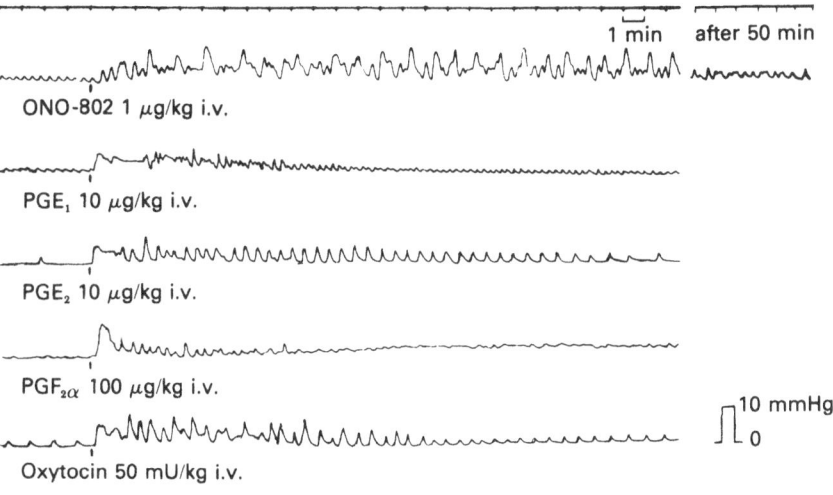

Figure 1.5   Effect of PGs and oxytocin on intrauterine pressure in the pregnant rat
(day 20)

The uterine stimulant potency of ONO-802 in rats on day 20 of
pregnancy after intravenous injection can be seen to be some ten times
greater than that of PGE_1 and PGE_2 and 100 times greater than $PGF_{2\alpha}$
(Figure 1.5). A single injection of ONO-802 (1 μg/kg i.v.) had a very
long-lasting uterine stimulant action. By comparison, PGE_1 and PGE_2
at 10 μg/kg i.v. produced uterine contractions of a comparable
magnitude but with a shorter duration of action. $PGF_{2\alpha}$, when
administered at the much larger dose of 100 μg/kg, again showed
relatively short, fading activity.

Intravenous injection of the same compound in pregnant Japanese
monkeys shows a very similar profile of activity. ONO-802 induces
long-lasting uterine contractions with an i.v. dose of just 0.1 μg/kg.
This response is equivalent to that produced by $PGF_{2\alpha}$ at an i.v. dose
of 20 μg/kg. Not only is ONO-802 two hundred times more potent than
$PGF_{2\alpha}$, it is also active vaginally. A vaginal dose of 10 μg/kg produced
tonic uterine contractions lasting about 3 hours, and the uterine
pressure was maintained at or around 40 mmHg during this period.
This last comment is quite an important one. Observations of the
response of this primate to uterine stimulation indicates that if the
pressure goes higher than this, the increased uterine contractions at
this higher pressure can be associated with pain. There is some
evidence that similar effects are seen in women.

As mentioned earlier, our search for a potent uterine stimulant was
based on the assumption that such activity would cause abortion at

9

Table 1.5   Abortifacient effect in Japanese monkeys with vaginal ONO-802

Monkey No.	Body weight (kg)	Stage of pregnancy (days)	Dose (µg/kg 3-hourly) and number of doses	Time of onset of bleeding (h)*	Duration of bleeding (days)	Time of fetal expulsion (h)*
1	8.8	27	Day 27 : 57 × 4	3	6	—
2	7.0	70	Day 70 : 50 × 3 Day 71 : 50 × 1	7	6	26.5
3	7.0	80	Day 80 : 20 × 4 Day 81 : 20 × 1	6	6	27.5
4	6.4	90	Day 90 : 20 × 4 Day 91 : 20 × 1	3	7	25
5	12.0	145	Day 145 : 20 × 4 Day 146 : 20 × 1	7	7	26

* From first treatment dose of ONO-802

various stages of pregnancy by a non-luteolytic mechanism. ONO-802 does, in fact, induce abortion in primates at various stages of pregnancy. In an experiment carried out by investigators at the Ono Pharmaceutical Company[20] and reported in Table 1.5[21], abortion was induced in five Japanese monkeys with pregnancies ranging from 27 to 145 days. The doses shown in the fourth column are in µg/kg administered intravaginally. Menstrual bleeding was induced in all five animals and the duration of bleeding was not abnormal. Products of conception were expelled in four of the animals. Much lower doses were required at later stages of pregnancy than at the earlier stages. Confirmation that abortion had been induced in animal No. 1 was obtained by an examination of the uterine size after treatment, by the observation of the onset of a normal menstruation subsequently, and by the pattern of hormonal changes observed in this monkey. Normal oestrus in the animal was characterized by increased progesterone secretion, which subsequently returned to a low level prior to menstruation. After mating, pregnancy of the animal was characterized by a much larger progesterone surge. The maintenance of that progesterone production is necessary for a viable pregnancy. On day 27 of pregnancy, ONO-802 was administered and a sharp decrease of progesterone followed, which coincided with the onset of menstrual bleeding and abortion. At a later stage, another surge of progesterone occurred, indicating normal oestrus, followed by a decrease in production of the hormone and the start of menstrual bleeding. Other studies carried out in Japan have shown, in a separate series of experiments in

Table 1.6 Chronic toxicity of ONO-802 in rodents

Species	Duration	Route and daily dose (μg/kg)	Comment
Rat ♀	1 month	Vaginal 10, 50, 250, 1250	Ten rats/group
			No toxicity
		6250	4/10 deaths
Rat ♀	26 week*	s.c. 2, 100	45 rats/group
			No toxicity
		250, 1000	No drug related deaths†

* With recovery at 4 and 13 weeks
† 28 rats died: 21 due to blood sampling; 3 were killed; 2 controls and 2 treated died. (250 and 1000 μg/kg)

monkeys, that ONO-802 produces a definite cervix-dilating effect following administration of vaginal pessaries containing 1 mg of ONO-802[22].

We at May & Baker and our colleagues at Ono have carried out extensive toxicology studies on ONO-802 in rodents and primates[23]. In rats, dosed daily for 1 month by the vaginal route (Table 1.6), no toxicity was noted at doses up to 1.25 mg/kg, although death occurred in four out of ten animals at the very high dose of 6.25 mg/kg. In a separate 26-week toxicity study involving subcutaneous dosing, no drug-related deaths were produced by the highest dose tested – 1 mg/kg. To put this in context, since the maximum therapeutic dose in women is 5 mg over a 12-hour period, which is approximately equivalent to 100 μg/kg, it is apparent that there is a good margin of safety.

Primates are probably the most suitable species for toxicity studies on drugs for human use. Because of the practical difficulties of administering exact vaginal doses to monkeys, Cynomolgus monkeys were dosed subcutaneously with ONO-802 (Table 1.7). Three dosages were chosen – 100, 300 and 750 μg/kg. The one mortality recorded was an animal killed on humane grounds following collapse after one of the doses although this was not apparently a dose-related effect[23]. Clinical signs at the highest doses included collapse, muscular trembling, unsteady posture, poorly formed faeces, excessive salivation and some local reaction at injection sites.

In an effort to obtain some evidence of vaginal toxicity and local tolerance, a small number of primates were dosed daily with a vaginal pessary containing 1 mg/kg for 27 days. No deaths were observed,

Table 1.7   ONO-802 one month toxicity study in the Cynomolgus monkey

Route:	s.c.
Dosage:	100, 300, 750 μg/kg
Mortalities:	1 monkey after a 300 μg/kg dose collapsed. Killed on humane grounds
Clinical signs (post-dosing)	Subdued behaviour
	Collapse (3 occasions)
	Muscular trembling (unsteady posture)
	Poorly formed faeces
	Excessive salivation
	Local reaction at injection sites

which again indicates a good margin of safety compared to the vaginal dose of up to 100 μg/kg administered over 12 hours, which would be administered to women.

SUMMARY

The pharmacological characteristics of ONO-802 are summarized in Table 1.8. ONO-802 produces strong uterine contractions which are long-lasting. The initial increase in contractility is a gradual one, which would be thought to minimize pain during use. It has good tissue selectivity, and the doses which are used to cause uterine contractions produce low side-effects of vomiting, nausea, diarrhoea. Its abortifacient effect is independent of ovarian function, meaning that it does not act by a luteolytic mechanism. I must stress that the cervix-dilating effect is a mechanism in its own right, it is not directly related to uterine contractions. Finally, the product is effective by the vaginal route. On the basis of this pharmacological evidence, both we at May & Baker and the Ono Pharmaceutical Co. embarked on a programme of clinical trials. Some of the results of these clinical trials will be presented at this Symposium by the clinicians who conducted them.

Table 1.8   ONO-802: Pharmacological characteristics

1. Strong uterine contractions
2. Long-lasting contractions
3. Gradual increase in contractility
4. Good tissue-selectivity
5. Abortifacient effect independent of ovarian function
6. Cervix-dilating effect
7. Vaginally effective

12

References

1 Mathé, A. A. (1977). Prostaglandins and the lung: Bronchopulmonary effects of prostaglandins. In Ramwell, P. W. (ed.) *The Prostaglandins*. (New York: Plenum Press)

2 Nakano, J. (1971). Relationship betwen the chemical structures of prostaglandins and their vasoactivities in dogs. *Pharmacologist*, **13**, 292

3 Samuelsson, B. (1963). Isolation and identification of prostaglandins from human seminal plasma. *J. Biol. Chem.*, **238**, 3229

4 Hamberg, M. and Samuelsson, B. (1966). Prostaglandins in human seminal plasma. *J. Biol. Chem.*, **241**, 257

5 Eglington, G., Raphael, R. A., Smith, G. N., Hall, W. J. and Pickles, V. R. (1963). The isolation and identification of two smooth muscle stimulants from menstrual fluid. *Nature (London)*, **200**, 993

6 Bygdeman, M. (1964). The effect of different prostaglandins on the human myometrium *in vitro*. *Acta Physiol. Scand.*, **63**, Suppl. 242, 1

7 Karim, S. M. M. (1966). Identification of prostaglandins in human amniotic fluid. *J. Obstet. Gynaecol. Br. Commonw.*, **73**, 230

8 Karim, S. M. M. (1967). The identification of prostaglandins in human umbilical cord. *Br. J. Pharmacol. Chemother.*, **29**, 230

9 Karim, S. M. M. (1968). Appearance of prostaglandin $F_{2\alpha}$ in human blood during labour. *Br. Med. J.*, **4**, 618

10 Kirton, K. T. (1975). Prostaglandins and reproduction in sub-human primates. In Karim, S. M. M. (ed.) *Advances in Prostaglandin Research. Prostaglandins and Reproduction*, pp. 229–270. (Lancaster: MTP Press)

11 Karim, S. M. M. and Hillier, K. (1975). Physiological roles and pharmacological actions of prostaglandins in relation to human reproduction. In Karim, S. M. M. (ed.) *Advances in Prostaglandin Research. Prostaglandins and Reproduction*, pp. 23–75. (Lancaster: MTP Press)

12 Sawyer, M. M., Lipshitz, J., Anderson, G. D. and Ditts, P. D. (1981). Third trimester uterine rupture with vaginal prostaglandin E_2. *Am. J. Obstet. Gynecol.*, **140**, 710

13 Ferreira, S. H. and Vane, J. R. (1967). Prostaglandins: Their disappearance from and release into the circulation. *Nature (London)*, **216**, 868

14 Anderson, G. G. and Speroff, L. (1973). Clinical use of prostaglandins in reproduction. In Ramwell, P. W. (ed.) *The Prostaglandins*. Vol. 1, pp. 365–389. (New York: Plenum Press)

15 Cooper, M. J. and Walpole, A. L. (1975). Practical applications of prostaglandins in animal husbandry. In Karim, S. M. M. (ed.) *Advances in Prostaglandin Research. Prostaglandins and Reproduction*, pp. 309–328. (Lancaster: MTP Press)

16 Csapo, A. I. and Mocsary, P. (1976). Menstrual induction by the vaginal application of ICI 81008 gel. *Prostaglandins*, **12**, 455

17 Pulkkinen, M. O. (1979). In Friebel, K., Schneider, A. and Würfel, H. (eds.) *International Sulprostone Symposium, Vienna, November 1978*, pp. 77–84. (Berlin: Schering AG Medico-Scientific Series)

18 Bygdeman, M., Gréen, K., Bergström, S., Bundy, G. and Kimball, F. (1979). New prostaglandin E analogue for pregnancy termination. *Lancet*, **1**, 1136

19 Bygdeman, M., Bremme, K., Christensen, N, Lundström, V. and Gréen, K. (1980). A comparison of two stable prostaglandin E analogues for termination of early pregnancy and for cervical dilatation. *Contraception*, **22**, 471

20 Oshima, K., Aso, T. and Hayashi, M. (1979). Uterine contractility and plasma levels of steroid hormones after intravaginal treatment of pregnant Japanese monkeys *(Macaca fuscata fuscata)* with 16,16-dimethyl-*trans*-Δ^2-prostaglandin E_1 methyl ester. *J. Reprod. Fertil.*, **55**, 353

21 Data on file, Ono Pharmaceutical Company
22 Oshima, K., Aso, T. and Tsuda, T. (1980). Effect of 16,16-dimethyl-*trans*-Δ^2 PGE$_1$ methyl ester (ONO-802) on cervical dilatation in pregnant monkeys. *Acta Obstet. Gynaecol. Japan*, **32**, 1038
23 Data on file, May & Baker Ltd

2
Clinical applications of prostaglandins in obstetrics and gynaecology

S. M. M. KARIM

INTRODUCTION

The use of prostaglandins in obstetrics and gynaecology is now firmly established. Most applications in this area are based on the ability of prostaglandins to modify the activity of the human uterus. This property was first recognized in 1930 and has since been confirmed by numerous investigators using pure prostaglandins.

It has also been established that endogenous prostaglandins are of physiological importance in regulating many reproductive functions. They are involved in ovulation, menstruation, spontaneous abortion, premature and term labour and in bringing about changes in the cervix that occur prior to the onset of labour. Most of the uses of exogenous prostaglandins in obstetrics and gynaecology are, thus, based on mimicking natural processes[1].

Practical applications of prostaglandins in obstetrics and gynaecology include:

(1) Menstrual induction/termination of very early pregnancy.

(2) Termination of first trimester pregnancy.

(3) Pre-evacuation cervical dilatation in first trimester of pregnancy.

(4) Termination of second trimester pregnancy.

15

(5) Termination of abnormal intra-uterine pregnancy.

(6) Pre-induction cervical ripening.

(7) Induction of labour.

(8) Control of post-partum haemorrhage.

(9) Post-partum and post-surgical retention of urine.

In addition drugs that inhibit the synthesis of prostaglandins have also found several useful applications in obstetrics and gynaecology. These include primary dysmenorrhoea, premature labour and irregular uterine bleeding.

Menstrual regulation

The importance of the corpus luteum in the normal menstrual cycle and in the maintenance of early pregnancy (up to 7th week from last menstrual period) is well established. There has always been an interest in drugs which might inhibit corpus luteum function since they could be used as postcoital contraceptives or early abortifacients to be taken once a month or only when there is a delay in menstruation (suggesting early pregnancy) of 2–3 weeks. Such drugs could also be used as an alternative to conventional contraceptives or to abortion performed later in pregnancy.

Prostaglandins (particularly $PGF_{2\alpha}$) have been shown to cause regression of the corpus luteum in several animal species[2-4], but so far it has not been possible to demonstrate convincingly that prostaglandins given in pharmacological doses produce corpus luteum regression in the human female[1,5].

In spite of a lack of direct effect of prostaglandins on the human corpus luteum, these compounds have been successfully used to induce menstruation when this is delayed by up to 2 weeks. Since the treatment is associated with a decrease in peripheral plasma progesterone, it may imply that prostaglandins are acting on the corpus luteum. This is likely to be an indirect effect resulting from strong uterine contractions disrupting the newly implanted blastocyst and thus removing the trophic influence on the corpus luteum. Menstrual induction has been attempted with prostaglandins given by intravenous, vaginal and intra-uterine routes.

NATURAL PROSTAGLANDINS

Vaginal administration of PGE_2 (up to 20 mg 2-hourly) or $PGF_{2\alpha}$ (up to 50 mg 2-hourly) for menstrual induction is not consistently effective and causes an unacceptably high incidence of side-effects which include severe uterine cramps, vomiting, diarrhoea and pyrexia. Similarly, inconsistent efficacy and high incidence of side-effects have been encountered when these two compounds are given by the intravenous route[6, 7]. More consistent results have been obtained when PGE_2 or $PGF_{2\alpha}$ is administered as a single intra-uterine dose but again the incidence of side-effects has been unacceptable.

SYNTHETIC ANALOGUES

The efficacy of several prostaglandin analogues administered by the vaginal and intra-uterine routes for menstrual induction has been explored in many clinical trials. The compounds studied include:

Compound	Route
15-methyl $PGF_{2\alpha}$ and its methyl ester	intra-uterine/vaginal
16-phenoxy-ω-tetranor PGE_2 methylsulfonylamide (Sulprostone)	intra-uterine
16,16-dimethyl PGE_2 and esters	vaginal
16,16-dimethyl-*trans*-Δ^2 PGE_1 methyl ester (Cervagem)	vaginal/intra-uterine

Results of some of these studies are summarized in Tables 2.1 and 2.2.

Studies with various prostaglandin analogues indicate that a high success rate with a low incidence of side-effects can be achieved with a single intra-uterine dose of some compounds. However, the procedure does not lend itself to self-administration which is a limiting factor in the widespread use of these compounds.

The simplicity of the vaginal route, and its potential for self-administration, can make this method an attractive alternative to surgical menstrual regulation. However, the incidence of side-effects with 15-methyl $PGF_{2\alpha}$ is very high. Results with 16,16-dimethyl-*trans*-Δ^2 PGE_1 methyl ester (Cervagem) are encouraging and further studies are being carried out to confirm the early findings.

Table 2.1   Results of menstrual induction with intra-uterine administration of prostaglandin analogues

Reference	No. of cases	Type of PG and dose	Success*	Side-effects
Ylikorkala et al. (1975)[23]	10	15-methyl $PGF_{2\alpha}$ 125 µg†	90%	nausea 40% vomiting 20% diarrhoea 40%
	10	200 µg†	70%	nausea 30% vomiting 30% diarrhoea 30%
	10	300 µg†	100%	nausea 39% vomiting 30% diarrhoea 20%
Karim et al. (1977)[24]	240	16-phenoxy-ω-tetranor PGE_2 methylsulfonylamide (Sulprostone) 50µg	95%	vomiting 5.4% headache 3.8% endometritis 0.8%
Tagaki et al. (1977)[25]	45	16,16-dimethyl-*trans*-Δ^2 PGE_1 methyl ester (ONO-802) 20–80 µg‡	93%	nausea 20% vomiting 16%

* Complete abortion
† Single dose
‡ More than 1 dose

TERMINATION OF FIRST TRIMESTER PREGNANCY

For the purpose of the present discussion only gestation of 7–12 weeks is included. Although prostaglandins have been successfully used for the termination of first trimester pregnancy, they compare less favourably with the vacuum aspiration method as the following comparison shows.

Comparison of vacuum aspiration and prostaglandins for termination of first trimester pregnancy:

Vacuum aspiration
(1) Can be performed within minutes.

(2) Can be performed in an outpatient clinic.

Prostaglandins
(1) Takes several hours.

(2) Requires overnight hospitalization of patients.

(3) Abortion is complete in more than 95% of the cases.

(3) Abortion is incomplete in more than 50% of the cases – vacuum aspiration or curettage necessary.

(4) Immediate side-effects minimal.

(4) Most patients experience uterine cramps, vomiting and diarrhoea.

(5) Necessary to dilate the cervix mechanically.

(5) No need to dilate the cervix.

Table 2.2   Results of menstrual induction with vaginal administration of prostaglandin analogues

No. of cases	Type of PG and dose	Success	Side-effects	Reference
38	15-methyl $PGF_{2\alpha}$ 2.0 mg × 1	76.3%	vomiting 37% diarrhoea 32%	Gréen et al. (1978)[26]
35	2.5 mg × 1	85.7%	vomiting 32% diarrhoea 51%	
128	3.0 mg × 1	94.5%	vomiting 54% diarrhoea 59%	
104	15-methyl $PGF_{2\alpha}$ 3.0 mg × 1	91.0%	vomiting 24% diarrhoea 37%	Mandelin (1978)[27]
50	16,16-dimethyl-trans-Δ^2 PGE_1 methyl ester (ONO-802) 1.0 mg × 5 doses	92.0%	vomiting 4% diarrhoea 6%	Karim et al. (1977)[28]
63	16,16-dimethyl-trans-Δ^2 PGE_1 methyl ester (ONO-802) 0.5 mg × 2 to 1.0 mg × 4	86.0%	vomiting 1.6% headache 4.8%	Tagaki et al. (1978)[29]
34	16,16-dimethyl-PGE_2 1.0 mg × 2–4 doses	100.0%	vomiting 26.5% diarrhoea 35.3%	Mackenzie et al. (1978)[30]

Pre-operative cervical dilatation with prostaglandins

The main disadvantage of termination of pregnancy by vacuum aspiration is the need to dilate mechanically the cervix in all nulliparae and most multiparae after the 10th week of gestation. Forceful dilatation may lead to damage to the cervix which results in a higher incidence of spontaneous abortion and premature labour in subsequent pregnancy.

Prostaglandins have a specific effect of softening and dilating the pregnant human cervix. This property has been utilized for achieving gradual cervical dilatation (and thus avoiding mechanical dilatation) in the first trimester of pregnancy prior to evacuation of the uterus by vacuum aspiration.

In order to make the use of prostaglandins for pre-evacuation cervical dilatation a practical one, it is necessary

(1)   to produce cervical dilatation in the shortest possible time to make outpatient termination possible;

(2)   to use a non-invasive (non-uterine) route;

(3)   that side-effects should be minimal.

Table 2.3   Pre-operative cervical dilatation in nulliparous women

No. of cases	Gestation weeks	PG/dose/route	Success	Side-effects	Reference
80	7–12	16-phenoxy-ω-17,18,19,20-tetranor PGE$_2$ methylsulfonylamide 0.5 mg i.m. (Sulprostone)	75%	Vomiting 5% Pyrexia 2.5% Uterine cramps 3%	Karim *et al.* (1978)[31]
180	6–13	16,16-dimethyl-*trans*-Δ^2 PGE$_1$ methyl ester 1 mg vaginal pessary (Cervagem)	80%	Nil	Prasad *et al.* (1978)[32]

The following prostaglandin analogues administered by the intramuscular and vaginal routes, 3–4 hours before evacuation of the uterus, produce adequate cervical dilatation to make evacuation of the uterus possible without mechanical dilatation of the cervix:

16,16-dimethyl-PGE$_2$ *p*-benzaldehyde semicarbazone ester (intramuscular/vaginal)
16-phenoxy-ω-tetranor-PGE$_2$ methylsulfonylamide (intramuscular)
16,16-dimethyl-*trans*-Δ^2 PGE$_1$ methyl ester (vaginal)

Results of some of the studies are shown in Table 2.3.

20

Table 2.4 Results of abortion with the use of intra-amniotic PGF$_{2\alpha}$ and 15-methyl PGF$_{2\alpha}$ from multicentre study*

Compound	Type of study	Dose (mg)	Total no. of patients	Success 24h No.	24h %	48h No.	48h %	Mean no. of episodes Vomiting	Diarrhoea	Cervical injury %	Complete abortion %
15-methyl PGF$_{2\alpha}$	Pilot study	2.5	311	238	76.4	296	95.2	1.9	0.7	NR§	49.0
PGF$_{2\alpha}$	Randomized	40	251	136	54.1	205	81.7†	1.5†	0.4‡	NR§	52.1
15-methyl PGF$_{2\alpha}$	Comparison	2.5	275	198	72.0	263	95.6†	2.1†	1.3‡		51.3
PGF$_{2\alpha}$	Randomized	50	351	238	67.8	304	86.6‡	1.3	0.5‡	2.9	55.3
15-methyl PGF$_{2\alpha}$	Comparison	2.5	333	247	74.1	309	92.8‡	1.7	1.2‡	2.9	55.3

* WHO (1977)[33]
† $p < 0.001$
‡ $p < 0.05$
§ NR = not reported

TERMINATION OF SECOND TRIMESTER PREGNANCY

Prostaglandins E_2, $F_{2\alpha}$ and several analogues administered by the intravenous, intramuscular, extra-amniotic, intra-amniotic and vaginal routes have been successfully used for the termination of second trimester pregnancy. There is a general agreement that some of the synthetic analogues have a more selective action on the uterus and are more effective in terminating second trimester pregnancy.

Intra-amniotic route

In several studies, 15-methyl $PGF_{2\alpha}$ in a single intra-amniotic dose of 2.5 mg has been used for the termination of second trimester pregnancy. Although the success rate (i.e. percentage of patients aborting in a given time) with this analogue has been higher than with 40 mg or 50 mg $PGF_{2\alpha}$ given intra-amniotically, the incidence of nausea, vomiting and diarrhoea was significantly higher in patients receiving 15-methyl $PGF_{2\alpha}$ (see Tables 2.4 and 2.5).

Table 2.5 Comparison of intra-amniotic $PGF_{2\alpha}$ (50 mg) and 15-methyl $PGF_{2\alpha}$ (2.5 mg) for the termination of second trimester pregnancy: results of a multicentre study

	$PGF_{2\alpha}$	15-methyl $PGF_{2\alpha}$
Number of patients	430	455
Dose	50 mg	2.5 mg
Success rate (48 h)	88.1%	93.0%
Induction–abortion interval (h)	19.2	19.3
Complete abortion	48.8%	56.0%
Blood loss > 500 ml	2.4%	1.4%
Vomiting (mean no. of episode/patient)	1.1	1.3
Diarrhoea (mean no. of episode/patient)	0.6	1.2
Cervical injury	4.7%	1.4%
Maternal death (number)	1	1

Data from Tejuja et al. (1978)[34]

Efficacy similar to that reported in the above studies can be achieved with a smaller dose of 15-methyl $PGF_{2\alpha}$[8, 9]. The use of a lower dose is associated with a considerably lower incidence of side-effects.

Extra-amniotic route

Administration of PGE_2 and $PGF_{2\alpha}$ by the extra-amniotic route for pregnancy termination usually involves repeated or continuous administration via an indwelling catheter. 15-methyl $PGF_{2\alpha}$ has a longer duration of action and the possibility of terminating second trimester pregnancy by the extra-amniotic route has been explored in a multicentre trial sponsored by the WHO Prostaglandin Task Force. The results are summarized in Table 2.6.

Table 2.6   Termination of pregnancy with a single extra-amniotic dose of 0.92 mg 15-methyl $PGF_{2\alpha}$ in Hyskon

	Number	%
Patients	600	100
Primigravidae	193	29.2
Multigravidae	467	70.8
Gestation (10–20 weeks)		
Fetus expelled		
24 h	479	72.6
30 h	509	77.1
36 h	530	80.3
Side-effects:		
Diarrhoea	212	32.2
Vomiting	246	37.7
Flushing	22	3.3
Chest pain	7	1.1
Blood loss > 500 ml	5	0.75
Cervical laceration	1	0.15

Data from WHO (1977)[35]

2a, 2b-dihomo-15-methyl $PGF_{2\alpha}$ methyl ester

This analogue in a single dose of 1 mg administered extra-amniotically produced abortion in 270 (85.4%) out of 316 patients within 24 h. Those who failed to abort were given a second dose or the uterus was evacuated by vacuum aspiration if the gestation was 14 weeks or below since the prostaglandin usually produced adequate cervical dilatation. The frequency of gastro-intestinal side-effects was significantly less than with 15-methyl $PGF_{2\alpha}$[9].

Intramuscular route

15-methyl $PGF_{2\alpha}$ administered intramuscularly has been used in many studies for termination of second trimester pregnancy. Results of selected studies are summarized in Table 2.7.

23

Table 2.7 Termination of pregnancy with intramuscular administration of 15(S)-15-methyl $PGF_{2\alpha}$

No. of cases	Gestation range weeks	Dose/schedule	Success rate (%)	Mean abortion time (h)	Side-effects*	Reference
30	15.2 (mean)	200–500 μg, 3-hourly	100	16.1	V: 4.7 episodes/patient D: 0.7 episodes/patient Flushing = 10	Bygdeman et al. (1974)[36]
80	8–22	350–500 μg, 2-hourly	100	15.7	V: 89%, D: 89%, P: 18%	Bolognese and Corson (1975)[37]
68	10–21	250 μg, 2-hourly	97	16.4	V: 79%, D: 86% Uterine rupture 1 case	Lange and Secher (1977)[38]
515	10–20	Initial dose 200 μg followed by 300 μg, 3-hourly	84.9	14.7	V: 2.9 episodes/patient D: 2.8 episodes/patient	WHO multicentre study (1977)[39]

V = Vomiting; D = diarrhoea; P = pyrexia
* Most patients premedicated with antidiarrhoeal before PG administration

Table 2.8 Results of termination of second trimester pregnancy with intramuscular injections of Sulprostone

| Group no. and dose of PG | No. of patients* | No. aborted | % aborted | Injection–abortion interval (hours mean and range) | | | Side-effects |
				Nulliparae	Multiparae	Whole group	
Group 1: 0.5 mg, 4-hourly	118	108	91.5	18.7 (7.25–36.0)	15.3 (3.5–36.0)	17.6 (3.5–36.0)	V = 29.6% D = 13.5% S = 13.5%
Group 2: 1.0 mg, 6-hourly	115	104	90.4	20.3 (5.0–36.0)	15.4 (2.5–34.0)	17.9 (2.5–36.0)	V = 38.2% D = 18.2% S = 10.4%
Group 3: 1.0 mg, 8-hourly	80	72	90.0	18.4 (5.0–36.0)	16.9 (3.25–36.0)	17.8 (3.25–36.0)	V = 38.7% D = 22.5% S = 6.25%

Data from Karim (1979)[10]
V = Vomiting; D = diarrhoea; S = shivering
* Approximately 60% of the patients were nulliparae

Table 2.9 Termination of pregnancy with a single long-acting vaginal suppository containing 15-methyl PGF$_{2\alpha}$ methyl ester

No. of cases	Gestation range (weeks)	Dose/schedule	Success rate (%)	Mean I/A interval (h)	Premedication	Side-effects and complications (%)	Complete abortion (%)	References
25	12–20	3–3.5 mg, single suppository	92*	12.4	Nil	V = 60; 1.7 episodes/patient D = 40; 0.7 episodes/patient H = 8	60.8	Bygdeman et al. (1977)[40]
39	8–19	3 mg, single suppository	87.2†	15.4	Antiemetic and antidiarrhoeal 1 h before prostaglandin and repeated as necessary	V = 46.1; 1.2 episodes/patient D = 48.7; 1.9 episodes/patient P = 10.2; R = 2.5	48.7	Ballard et al. (1978)[41]
58	10–14	3 mg, single suppository	72.4‡	17.9	Lomotil 5 mg at 0, 3, 6 h	V = 0.8 episodes/patient D = 1.4 episodes/patient	NS	Kinra et al. (1978)[42]
50	12–20	2 mg, single suppository	78*	17.9	Lomotil 5 mg at 0, 3, 6 h	V = 3.2 episodes/patient D = 2.5 episodes/patient F = 18; R = 36; P = 16	NS	Mandelin and Kajanoja (1978)[43]

V = Vomiting; D = diarrhoea; H = haemorrhage (>500 ml); P = pyrexia; F = flushing; R = rigors; NS = not stated

* = Fetus expelled within 24 h
† = Fetus expelled within 27 h
‡ = Fetus expelled within 30 h

While there is no doubt about the efficacy of 15-methyl $PGF_{2\alpha}$ given by the intramuscular route for termination of second trimester pregnancy, the incidence of vomiting and diarrhoea is too high (in spite of pre-medication to counteract these side-effects) for routine use of this compound.

16-phenoxy-ω-17,18,19,20-tetranor PGE_2 methylsulfonylamide (Sulprostone)

This analogue, given by different intramuscular doses, has been used in several studies. Results of one such study involving 313 patients are shown in Table 2.8[10].

Vaginal route

Considerable efforts have been put into developing a single long-acting vaginal suppository for termination of second trimester pregnancy. Results of some studies are shown in Table 2.9.

CERVICAL TEAR AND UTERINE RUPTURE

The most serious complication of prostaglandin-induced abortion is cervical injury. This is probably the result of unusual cervical resistance in the face of strong uterine contractions and therefore is more likely to occur in young nulliparae in the late second trimester of pregnancy. The incidence of cervical tear is difficult to assess but when reported[11] it has ranged between 0.3% and 8%.

COMBINATION WITH LAMINARIA

It has been suggested that insertion of one or more laminaria tents into the cervical canal a few hours before prostaglandin administration may prevent cervical rupture. In practice, such a procedure also significantly reduced abortion interval[12](see Table 2.10 for results).

TERMINATION OF ABNORMAL INTRA-UTERINE PREGNANCY

The successful use of prostaglandin E_2 infusion at the rate of 5 μg/min to terminate abnormal intra-uterine pregnancies (missed abortion, intra-uterine fetal death, and molar pregnancy) was first reported by Karim in 1970. Since then PGE_2 and $PGF_{2\alpha}$ given by several different

Table 2.10 Results of termination of pregnancy with laminaria and Sulprostone

Group no. and treatment	Fetus expelled in 30 h						Injection–abortion interval (Hours, mean and range)		
	Nulliparae		Multiparae		Total		Nulliparae	Multiparae	Whole group
	No.	%	No.	%	No.	%			
Group 1* Laminaria and Sulprostone, 1 mg 8-hourly	16/16	100.0	13/14	92.8	29/30	96.6	12.8†	7.3†	10.4†
Group 2 Sulprostone, 1 mg 8-hourly	17/20	85.0	9/10	90.0	26/30	86.7	18.8†	12.9†	16.7†
Group 3* Laminaria and Sulprostone, 0.5 mg 4-hourly	18/18	100.0	12/12	100.0	30/30	100.0	11.2‡	11.3‡	11.2‡
Group Sulprostone, 0.5 mg 4-hourly	15/19	78.9	11/11	100.0	26/30	86.7	19.8‡	14.4‡	17.5‡

Data from Karim et al. (1982)[12]
* A medium size laminaria was inserted 8 h before the first dose of Sulprostone
† $p < 0.001$ (Group 1 vs 2)
‡ $p < 0.01$ (Group 3 vs 4)

routes (intravenous, vaginal, intra-amniotic, extra-amniotic) have been shown to be effective in the same or smaller doses than those required for interruption of viable second trimester pregnancy[13].

Although intra-amniotic injection is generally accompanied by fewer side-effects, severe reactions have been described; these were probably due to an accelerated passage of the prostaglandins through the altered fetal membranes. In addition administration of a prostaglandin by the intra-uterine route may introduce an infection in the presence of a dead fetus.

Vaginal pessaries containing 20 mg PGE_2 administered at varying intervals have given good results in the termination of abnormal intra-uterine pregnancy but the incidence of side-effects has been high[13, 14].

2a,2b-dihomo-15(S)-15-methyl $PGF_{2\alpha}$ methyl ester, 15-methyl $PGF_{2\alpha}$ and 16-phenoxy-ω-tetranor PGE_2 methylsulfonylamide injected intramuscularly have proved very effective for termination of pregnancy in cases of intra-uterine fetal death, missed abortion and molar and anencephalic pregnancies[13–15]. Results of selected studies are shown in Table 2.11.

PRE-INDUCTION CERVICAL RIPENING

The outcome of attempted induction of labour at or near term depends on the state of the cervix. There is evidence to suggest that endogenous prostaglandin plays a role in cervical ripening at term. In some clinical situations the cervix remains unfavourable because the normal ripening process has failed to occur.

Prostaglandin E_2 administered by the intravenous, extra-amniotic, vaginal and oral routes has been shown to ripen an unfavourable cervix and thus improve the outcome of subsequent induction. The subject has been reviewed in detail by Calder[16].

Induction of labour

Prostaglandin E_2 given by the oral route has been used for the induction of labour at term in a large number of clinical trials. The results of these studies indicate that induction with oral PGE_2 combined with amniotomy is likely to be successful in the majority of multigravidae regardless of the state of the cervix. In primigravidae, however, successful outcome depends upon the state of the cervix. Failure rates in patients with an unfavourable cervix (Bishop Score 5 or below) are in the region of 15–20% but this figure can be reduced by pre-induction priming of the cervix as discussed above[17].

Table 2.11 Results of termination of abnormal intrauterine pregnancy with intramuscular administration of prostaglandin analogues

No. and type of cases	Success	Prostaglandin, dose	Mean expulsion interval (Average no. of injections)	Side-effects	Reference
63 MP: 9 MA: 30 IUD: 19 AP: 5	61 (96.8%) within 24 h	16-phenoxy-ω-tetranor PGE$_2$ methylsulfonylamide (Sulprostone), 0.5 mg, 6-hourly	9.5 h (2.0)	GI: 21% S: 6.3%	Karim et al. (1978)[44]
97 MA and IUD	96 (98.9%) within 30.5 h	15(S)-15-methyl PGF$_{2\alpha}$, 0.125–0.25 mg, 2-hourly	1.2–30.5 h (range) (Median 5.0)	GI: 89%	Wallenberg et al. (1980)[15]
631 MP: 82 MA 233 IUD: 282 AP: 34	600 (95.1%) within 32 h	2a,2b-dihomo-15(S)-15-methyl PGF$_{2\alpha}$ methyl ester, 0.5 mg, 8-hourly	11.3 h (1.8)	GI: 48% S: 11.9%	Karim et al. (1982)[45]

MP = Molar pregnancy; MA = Missed abortion; IUD = Intrauterine death; AP = Anencephalic pregnancy; GI = Gastrointestinal; S = Shivering

Post-partum haemorrhage

The use of prostaglandins in the management of post-partum haemorrhage remains almost unexplored. Reports from isolated cases indicate that these substances can control post-partum bleeding when conventional treatment has failed[18, 19]. Some prostaglandins given prophylactically after delivery have been shown to reduce post-partum blood loss[10, 20].

Post-partum and post-surgical retention of urine

Prostaglandin E_2 and $PGF_{2\alpha}$ are known to contract human bladder. In preliminary studies these compounds administered via a bladder catheter have proved useful in the management of urinary retention[21, 22].

References

1 Karim, S. M. M. and Hillier, K. (1975). Physiological roles and pharmacological actions of prostaglandins in relation to human reproduction. In Karim, S. M. M. (ed.) *Advances in Prostaglandin Research. Prostaglandins and Reproduction*, pp. 23–75. (Lancaster: MTP Press)

2 Labhsetwar, A. P. (1975). Prostaglandins and studies related to reproduction in laboratory animals. In *Advances in Prostaglandin Research. Prostaglandins and Reproduction*, pp. 241–270. Karim, S. M. M. (ed.) (Lancaster: MTP Press)

3 Kirton, K. T. (1975). Prostaglandins and Reproduction in sub-human primates. In Karim, S. M. M. (ed.) *Advances in Prostaglandin Research. Prostaglandins and Reproduction*, pp. 220–240. (Lancaster: MTP Press)

4 Cooper, M. J., Hammond, D. and Schultz, R. H. (1979). Veterinary uses of prostaglandins. In Karim, S. M. M. (ed.) *Advances in Prostaglandin Research. Practical Applications of Prostaglandins and their Synthesis Inhibitors*, pp. 189–216. (Lancaster: MTP Press)

5 Karim, S. M. M. and Rao, B. (1976). Prostaglandins in human reproduction. In Karim, S. M. M. (ed.) *Obstetric and Gynaecological Uses of Prostaglandin. Proceedings of Asian Federation of Obstetrics and Gynaecology 1st Inter-Congress, Singapore, April 1976*, pp. 1–21. (Lancaster: MTP Press)

6 Karim, S. M. M. and Amy, J. J. (1975). Interruption of pregnancy with prostaglandins. In Karim, S. M. M. (ed.) *Advances in Prostaglandin Research. Prostaglandins and Reproduction*, pp. 77–148. (Lancaster: MTP Press)

7 Bygdeman, M. (1979). Menstrual regulation with prostaglandins. In Karim, S. M. M. (ed.) *Advances in Prostaglandin Research. Practical Application of Prostaglandins and their Synthesis Inhibitors*, pp. 267–282. (Lancaster: MTP Press)

8 Karim, S. M. M. and Sivasamboo, R. (1975). Termination of second trimester pregnancy with intra-amniotic 15(S)15-methyl prostaglandin $F_{2\alpha}$ – A two dose schedule study. *Prostaglandins*, **9**, 487

9 Karim, S. M. M. (1976). Singapore experience with prostaglandins. In Karim, S. M. M. (ed.) *Obstetric and Gynaecological Uses of Prostaglandin. Proceedings of Asian Federation of Obstetrics and Gynaecology 1st Inter-Congress, Singapore, April 1976*, pp. 127–154. (Lancaster: MTP Press)

10 Karim, S. M. M. (1979). Prostaglandins in obstetrics and gynaecology. In Friebel, K., Schneider, A. and Wurfel, H. (eds.) *International Sulprostone Symposium, Vienna, November 1978*, pp. 7–28. (Berlin: Schering AG, Medico-Scientific Series)

11 Karim, S. M. M. (1979). Termination of second trimester pregnancy with prostaglandins. In Karim, S. M. M. (ed.) *Advances in Prostaglandin Research. Practical Applications of Prostaglandins and their Synthesis Inhibitors*, pp. 375–409. (Lancaster: MTP Press)

12 Karim, S. M. M., Ratnam, S. S., Lim, A. L., Yeo, K. C. and Choo, H. T. (1982). Termination of second trimester pregnancy with laminaria and intramuscular 16-phenoxy-ω-17,18,19,20-tetranor PGE_2 methylsulfonylamide (Sulprostone) – A randomized study. *Prostaglandins*, **23**, 257

13 Karim, S. M. M., Ng, S. S. and Ratnam, S. S. (1979) Termination of abnormal intrauterine pregnancy with prostaglandins. In Karim, S. M. M. (ed.) *Advances in Prostaglandin Research. Practical Applications of Prostaglandins and their Synthesis Inhibitors*, pp. 319–374. (Lancaster: MTP Press)

14 Southern, E. M., Gutknecht, G. D., Mohberg, N. R. and Edelman, D. A. (1978). Vaginal prostaglandin E_2 in the management of fetal intrauterine death. *Br. J. Obstet. Gynaecol.*, **85**, 437

15 Wallenberg, H. S. G., Keirse, M. J. N. C., Freie, H. M. P. and Blacquiere, J. F. (1980). Intramuscular administration of 15(S)15-methyl prostaglandin $F_{2\alpha}$ for induction of labour in patients with fetal death. *Br. J. Obstet. Gynaecol.*, **87**, 203

16 Calder, A. A. (1979). Prostaglandins for pre-induction cervical ripening. In Karim, S. M. M. (ed.) *Advances in Prostaglandin Research. Practical Application of Prostaglandins and their Synthesis Inhibitors*, pp. 301–318. (Lancaster: MTP Press)

17 Amy, J. J. and Thiery, M. (1979). Induction of labour with prostaglandins. In Karim, S. M. M. (ed.) *Advances in Prostaglandin Research. Practical Applications of Prostaglandins and their Synthesis Inhibitors*, pp. 437–446. (Lancaster: MTP Press)

18 Takagi, S., Yoshida, T., Yogo, T., Abe, M., Tochigi, H., Sakata, H. and Takahashi, H. (1976). The effects of uterine intramuscular injection of $PGF_{2\alpha}$ on severe post-partum haemorrhage. In Samuelsson, B. and Paoletti, R. (eds.) *Advances in Prostaglandin and Thromboxane Research*. Vol. 2, p. 1003. (New York: Raven Press)

19 Zahradnik, H. P., Steiner, H., Hillemanns, H. G., Breckwoldt, M. and Ardelt, W. (1977). Prostaglandin $F_{2\alpha}$ und 15-methyl prostaglandin $F_{2\alpha}$ Anwendung bei massiven uterinen Blatungen. *Geburtsh. Frauenheilk*, **37**, 493

20 Persianinov, L. S., Manuilova, I. A. and Chernukha, E. A. (1973). The result of using prostaglandin $F_{2\alpha}$ for induction and stimulation of labor. In Bergström, S. and Bernhard, S. (eds.) *Advances in Biosciences*, **9**, pp. 585–592. (New York: Vieweg, Pergamon Press)

21 Bultitude, M. T., Hills, N. H. and Shuttleworth, K. E. D. (1976). Clinical and experimental studies on the action of prostaglandins and their synthesis inhibitors on detrusor muscle in vitro and in vivo. *Br. J. Urol.*, **48**, 631

22 Ratnam, S. S., Prasad, R. N. V. and Karim, S. M. M. (1979). Management of post-surgical urinary retention with prostaglandin $F_{2\alpha}$. A preliminary report. *Singapore J. Obstet. Gynaecol.*, **10**, 23

23 Ylikorkala, O., Kirkinen, P., Jouppila, P. and Jarvinen, P. A. (1975). Intrauterine injection of 15(S)15-methyl prostaglandin $F_{2\alpha}$ for termination of early pregnancy in out patient. *Prostaglandins*, **10**, 333

24 Karim, S. M. M., Rao B., Ratnam, S. S., Prasad, R. N. V., Wong, Y. M. and Illancheran, A. (1977). Termination of early pregnancy (menstrual induction) with 16-phenoxy-ω-tetranor PGE_2 methylsulfonylamide. *Contraception*, **16**, 377

25 Takagi, S., Sakata, H., Yoshida, T. *et al.* (1977). Termination of very early pregnancy by ONO-802 (16,16-dimethyl-trans-Δ^2-PGE_1 methyl ester). *Prostaglandins*, **14**, 791

26 Gréen, K., Bygdeman, M. and Bremme, K. (1978). Interruption of early first trimester pregnancy by single vaginal administration of 15-methyl-PGF$_{2\alpha}$ methyl ester. *Contraception*, **18**, 551

27 Mandelin, M. (1978). Termination of early pregnancy by a single dose 3 mg 15-methyl PGF$_{2\alpha}$ methyl ester vaginal suppository. *Prostaglandins*, **16**, 143

28 Karim, S. M. M., Ratnam, S. S. and Illancheran, A. (1977). Menstrual induction with vaginal administration of 16,16-dimethyl-trans-Δ^2 PGE$_1$ methyl ester (ONO-802). *Prostaglandins*, **14**, 615

29 Takagi, S., Sakata, H., Yoshida, T. *et al.* (1978). Termination of early pregnancy by ONO-802 suppositories (16,16-dimethyl-trans-Δ^2 PGE$_1$ methyl ester). *Prostaglandins*, **15**, 913

30 Mackenzie, I. A., Embrey, M. P., Davies, P. and Guillebaud, J. (1978). Very early abortion by prostaglandins. *Lancet*, **1**, 1223

31 Karim, S. M. M., Illancheran, A., Wun, W., Ho, T. H. and Ratnam, S. S. (1978). Intramuscular administration of 16-phenoxy-ω-17,18,19,20-tetranor PGE$_2$ methylsulfonylamide for pre-operative cervical dilatation in first trimester nulliparae. *Prostagl. Med.*, **1**, 71

32 Prasad, R. N. V., Lim, C., Wong, Y. C., Karim, S. M. M. and Ratnam, S. S. (1978). Vaginal administration of 16,16-dimethyl-trans-Δ^2 PGE$_1$ methyl ester (ONO-802) for pre-operative cervical dilatation in first trimester nulliparous pregnancy. *Singapore J. Obstet. Gynaecol.*, **9**, 69

33 WHO Task Force on the Use of Prostaglandins for the Regulation of Fertility (1977). Prostaglandins and abortion III. Comparison of single intra-amniotic injection of 15-methyl prostaglandin F$_{2\alpha}$ and prostaglandin F$_{2\alpha}$ for termination of second trimester pregnancy: An international multicentric study. *Am. J. Obstet. Gynecol.*, **129**, 601

34 Tejuja, S., Choudhury, S. D. and Manchanda, P. K. (1978). Use of intra- and extra-amniotic prostaglandins for the termination of pregnancies – Report of multicentric trial in India. *Contraception*, **18**, 641

35 WHO Task Force on the Use of Prostaglandins for the Regulation of Fertility (1977). Prostaglandins and abortion II. Single extra-amniotic administration of 0.92 mg of 15-methyl prostaglandin F$_{2\alpha}$ in Hyskon for termination of pregnancies in weeks 10 to 20 of gestation: An international multicentric study. *Am. J. Obstet. Gynecol.*, **129**, 597

36 Bygdeman, M., Martin, J. N., Wiqvist, N., Gréen, K. and Bergström, S. (1974). Reassessment of systemic administration of prostaglandins for induction of mid-trimester abortion. *Prostaglandins*, **8**, 157

37 Bolognese, R. J. and Corson, S. L. (1975). Interruption of pregnancy by prostaglandin 15-methyl F$_{2\alpha}$. *Fertil. Steril.*, **26**, 695

38 Lange, A. P. and Secher, J. J. (1977). Mid-trimester and missed abortion treated with intramuscular 15(S)15-methyl PGF$_{2\alpha}$. *Prostaglandins*, **14**, 389

39 WHO Task Force on the Use of Prostaglandins for the Regulation of Fertility (1977). Prostaglandins and abortion I. Intramuscular administration of 15-methyl prostaglandin F$_{2\alpha}$ for induction of abortion in weeks 10 to 20 of pregnancy. *Am. J. Obstet. Gynecol.*, **129**, 593

40 Bygdeman, M., Gangul, A., Kinoshita, K., Lundström, V., Gréen, K. and Bergström, S. (1977). Development of a vaginal suppository suitable for single administration for interruption of second trimester pregnancy. *Contraception*, **15**, 129

41 Ballard, C. A., Forte, K. Lauersen, N. H. (1978). Plasma prostaglandin concentration and abortifacient effectiveness of a single insertion of a 3 mg 15(S)15-methyl prostaglandin F$_{2\alpha}$ methyl ester vaginal suppository. *Contraception*, **17**, 383

42 Kinra, G., Agarwal, N., Jagannath, K. T. and Hingorani, V. (1978). Evaluation of a single dose schedule of 15(S)15-methyl PGF$_{2\alpha}$ methyl ester suppository for termination of 10–14 weeks of pregnancy. *Contraception*, **17**, 455

43 Mandelin, M. and Kajanoja, P. (1978). Induction of second trimester abortion. Comparison between vaginal 15-methyl PGF$_{2\alpha}$ methyl ester and intra-amniotic PGF$_{2\alpha}$. *Prostaglandins*, **16**, 995

44 Karim, S. M. M., Lim, A. L., Prasad, R. N. V., Yeo, K. C., Ng, S. C., Salmon, Y. M., Choo, H. T. and Ratnam, S. S. (1979). Termination of abnormal intrauterine pregnancy with intramuscular administration of Sulprostone. *Singapore J. Obstet. Gynaecol.*, **10**, 33

45 Karim, S. M. M., Ratnam, S. S., Hutabarat, H., Hanafiah, J., Simanjuntak, P., Teoh, S. K., Ong, S. K., Sen, D. K. and Sinathuray, T. A. (1982). Termination of pregnancy in cases of intrauterine fetal death, missed abortion, molar and anencephalic pregnancy with intravascular administration of 2a,2b-dihomo 15(S)15-methyl PGF$_{2\alpha}$ methyl ester – a multicenter study. *Ann. Acad. Med. Singapore*, **11**, 508

Discussion 1

(1) **Dr Lim Su Min** (Singapore): Is there a place for the use of prostaglandins in the non-pregnant uterus? I am specifically considering diagnostic curettage in infertile women. Sometimes the cervix is very firm and fibrous and may lacerate during attempt at instrumental dilatation. Can prostaglandins solve this problem?

Dr Karim (Singapore): Yes, with a qualification. Very few studies have been carried out to specifically answer this question. From time to time, I have been approached by obstetricians and gynaecologists in the hospital where I work and by some in private practice when they have tried to dilate the non-pregnant cervix and have failed to do so. We have supplied prostaglandins to these people and the reports that have come back indicate that the drug has been useful. So the answer to your question, Su Min, is 'yes'. Perhaps Professor Bygdeman would like to comment.

Dr Bygdeman (Sweden): Preoperative cervical dilatation induced by prostaglandins during pregnancy is most likely due to stimulation of uterine contractility pushing the conceptus through the cervical canal, and to a local effect on the cervix. When

35

treating the non-pregnant patient you have to rely only on the local effect. In summary, I am less impressed with the effect of PGs on the non-pregnant cervix as compared to the pregnant one.

(2) **Dr Sivasamboo** (Singapore): What is the mechanism of action of prostaglandins?

Dr Crowshaw (UK): Are you referring to the application that has been discussed today or do you mean in general? [Answer: in general]. The effect on the cervix seems to be basically a biochemical event. The PGs actually change the constituents in the cervix, particularly the collagen matrix, and this contributes to the cervical dilatation. As many of you are aware, it is not simply a relaxation of muscles associated with the cervix which causes cervical dilatation. There has been a symposium on the cervix and cervical dilatation very recently and a book has been published. In terms of the effects of PGs on the contractile effect on uterine smooth muscle, quite a bit is known but we cannot go into it today, but calcium is obviously very important as are cyclic AMP changes.

Dr Karim: My comments will be restricted to the mechanism of oxytocic effect of prostaglandins. There are recent studies which indicate a very close link between PGs and oxytocin and this mechanism would be relevant in the pregnant state. One of the properties of PGs, that is not widely known, is that most of the PGs that are effective in stimulating the uterus during pregnancy are potent inhibitors of the enzyme oxytocinase. They can thus build up the levels of oxytocin in circulation. There are studies which show exactly the opposite – oxytocin releasing PGs. Cyclic AMP and GMP are also thought to be involved. Thus we are dealing with a complex mechanism involving several potent biologically active substances.

(3) **Dr Phuaradit** (Thailand): Does Cervagem affect the bronchial smooth muscle?

Dr Crowshaw: We have not seen and we have had no reports of any bronchial effects of Cervagem after administration in clinical trials. PGEs are thought to be bronchodilators but the situation is more complex. PGE_2 can also produce bronchoconstriction. For that reason, we do put in all our clinical trial programmes a warning to look out for bronchial effects and a contraindication for use in patients with known history of problems involving the respiratory system. However, I must re-emphasize that we have seen no such reports to my knowledge in any of the clinical trials. Perhaps Professor Karim would like to comment.

Dr Karim: Not with Cervagem, but I have seen this with other PGs. $PGF_{2\alpha}$ is a bronchoconstrictor in sensitive subjects. You can give a healthy subject $500\,\mu g$ of $PGF_{2\alpha}$ intravenously. There is no bronchoconstriction. If you give as little as $10\,\mu g$ to a sensitive subject, an asthmatic, with a previous history of sensitivity, it is likely to produce bronchoconstriction. However, PG-induced broncho-constriction is easily reversible by conventional treatment. Any time there is a patient with a history of asthma, we tell the physician who is looking after her to have a bronchodilator available – salbutamol aerosol is very effective. So PG-induced bronchoconstriction is easily reversible but it is necessary to identify susceptible patients and give treatment immediately. It is also important to realize that some PGE analogues are extremely potent broncho-constrictors.

(4) **Dr Simandjuntak** (Indonesia): Is there any adverse reaction of synthetic PG analogues on live fetus? Is the efficacy of synthetic PG analogues lower when used to terminate a viable pregnancy compared to when used to evacuate a uterus with a dead fetus?

Dr Karim: Cervagem has only been used for termination of first and second trimester pregnancy. As I mentioned earlier, none of the synthetic analogues of PGs have been used or are likely to be used in the foreseeable future for induction of labour with the idea of bringing out a live fetus. So adverse reaction to the fetus is not known but is anticipated.

Generally speaking, a pregnancy with a dead fetus is a lot easier to terminate than a viable pregnancy at the corresponding stage of gestation.

Dr Crowshaw: I just might expand on that. The actual dose of PG required to terminate a pregnancy with a dead fetus is relatively low. The dose that we have been using in our clinical trials for termination of viable pregnancy with Cervagem is 1 mg (pessary) so the first point is that this would be far too high a dose anyway, and the second point that Professor Karim made was that we have no data whatsover to support the use of Cervagem for induction of labour at term. Many problems are anticipated. The first is uterine hypertonus and the other is that PGs do have effects on the fetus itself, on the live baby, including effects on the ductus and other structures. These could be life-threatening. The only prostaglandins used for induction of term labour are PGE_2 and $PGF_{2\alpha}$, both natural compounds. These have been found to be safe. Analogues of PGs have so far not been used for induction of term labour in the presence of a live fetus.

3
Pre-operative cervical dilatation: comparative study of Cervagem* and Sulprostone* in first trimester abortion

P. FYLLING and F. JERVE

INTRODUCTION

The use of prostaglandins (PGs) for pre-operative cervical dilatation prior to terminating late first trimester pregnancy, especially in primigravidae, is reported to be a methodological improvement[1-7].

For obvious reasons many departments are forced to perform therapeutic abortions on outpatient basis and treatment requiring overnight hospital stay can therefore be a disadvantage. A short pre-treatment period of 3–4 h, however, can easily be included in the time schedule for outpatient treatment. In addition, a simple route of administration will allow the patient herself or the nursing staff to administer the treatment.

Both Cervagem and Sulprostone are reported to induce sufficient cervical dilatation within a few hours of administration[4, 6-7]. The aim of the present study was to compare these two analogues with regard to efficacy and incidence of side-effects.

MATERIALS AND METHODS

One hundred and ten primigravidae, 9–12 weeks pregnant, with approval for legal abortion were selected at random into two groups:

*Cervagem: 16,16-dimethyl-*trans*-Δ_2 PGE$_1$ methyl ester; Sulprostone: 16-phenoxy-ω-17,18,19,20-tetranor PGE$_2$ methylsulfonylamide

Group I: 55 patients received a single intramuscular injection of 300 µg Sulprostone (Schering).

Group II: 55 patients received one vaginal pessary containing 1 mg Cervagem (ONO-802).

The patients were admitted at 0730 in fasting condition and both compounds were given 3–4 h prior to vacuum aspiration without additional premedication. The dilating effect on the cervix was estimated with Hegar dilators and the size of the largest dilator passing through the cervical canal without resistance was recorded. Following surgery the patients were kept in bed for 2–3 h and then discharged. A follow-up visit was arranged about 4 weeks later.

RESULTS

Both groups were similar concerning age and gestational length (Table 3.1). As seen from Table 3.2 a cervical dilatation of Hegar $\geqslant 7$ was achieved in 80 % of the women in the Cervagem group compared with 62 % in the Sulprostone group. No clinical effect was recorded in 7.3 % in the Sulprostone group compared with none in the Cervagem group.

The incidence of gastro-intestinal side-effects was negligible in both groups as shown in Table 3.3. Only one of the women in the Cervagem group and six in the Sulprostone group had one or more episodes of vomiting. Three women in the Cervagem group had diarrhoea and none in the Sulprostone group.

Table 3.1   Material – all primigravidae

	No.	Age (y)	Gest. length (weeks)
Cervagem	55	16–30 $\bar{x} = 21.6$	9–11 $\bar{x} = 10.2$
Sulprostone	55	16–42 $\bar{x} = 21.9$	9–11 $\bar{x} = 10.1$

Table 3.2   Cervical dilatation. Largest Hegar passing without resistance

	0–4	5–6	7–8	9–11
Cervagem	0.0%	20.0%	43.6%	36.4%
Sulprostone	7.3%	30.8%	45.5%	16.4%

Table 3.3   Gastro-intestinal side-effects

	Vomiting	Diarrhoea
Cervagem	1 (2%)	3 (5%)
Sulprostone	6 (11%)	0 (0%)

Table 3.4   Pain

	None	Slight	Moderate
Cervagem	16	34	5
Sulprostone	9	41	5

Two patients in each group received pethidine

As shown in Table 3.4 most of the women experienced only slight uterine pain and as many as 25 (22.7%) of them felt no pain and only four needed analgesia. There were no other side-effects associated with the medication.

DISCUSSION

Sufficient cervical dilatation was achieved in most of the patients within 3–4 h and the pre-treatment was associated with no or negligible side-effects. Although intramuscular administration is simple and can be handled by the nursing staff, vaginal pessaries are even more convenient and allow self-administration. Whether both compounds were given in optimal doses cannot be established from the present study. In previous studies (to be published) we have found that there may be a threshold with regard to gastro-intestinal side-effects with Sulprostone when given intramuscularly in doses between $300\,\mu g$ and $500\,\mu g$.

Pre-operative dilatation may reduce cervical damage[8,9]. Hence, in our opinion pretreatment with PGs should be advocated at least when terminating first trimester pregnancy in primigravidae.

ACKNOWLEDGEMENT

The study has been supported by Rhône-Poulenc/May & Baker Ltd and Schering AG.

References

1 Bygdeman, M., Bremme, K., Christensen, N., Lundström, V. and Gréen, K. (1980). A comparison of two stable prostaglandin E analogues for termination of early pregnancy and for cervical dilatation. *Contraception*, **22**, 471

2 Jerve, F. and Fylling, P. (1978). Therapeutic abortion in late first trimester. Prostaglandin pretreatment compared with primary surgery. *Prostgl. Med.*, **1**, 333

3 Karim, S. M. M., Choo, H. T. and Cheng, P. (1975). Cervical dilatation with prostaglandin analogues prior to vaginal termination of first pregnancy in nulliparous women. *Prostaglandins*, **9**, 631

4 Karim, S. M. M., Illancheran, A., Wun, W., Ho, T. H. and Ratnam, S. S. (1978). Vaginal administration of 16,16-phenoxy-ω-17,18,19,20-tetranor PGE$_2$ methyl-sulfonylamide for preoperative cervical dilatation in first trimester nulliparae. *Prostgl. Med.*, **1**, 71

5 Prasad, R. N. V., Lim, C., Wong, Y. C., Karim, S. M. M. and Ratnam, S. S. (1978). Vaginal administration of 16,16-dimethyl-trans-Δ^2 PGE$_1$ methyl ester (ONO-802) for preoperative cervical dilatation in first trimester nulliparous pregnancy. *Singapore J. Obstet. Gynaecol.*, **9**, 69

6 Wagatsuma, T., Tabuchi, T., Tabei, T. and Kaku, R. (1979). Interruption of pregnancy with vaginal suppositories containing 16,16-dimethyl-trans-Δ^2-prostaglandin E$_1$ methyl ester. *Contraception*, **19**, 591

7 WHO Task Force on Prostaglandins (1981). Vaginal administration of 15-methyl PGF$_{2\alpha}$ methyl ester for preoperative cervical dilatation. *Contraception*, **23**, 351

8 Edström, K. B. (1975). Early complications and late sequelae of induced abortion. A review of the literature. *Bull. WHO*, **52**, 123

9 Johnstone, F. D., Beard, R., Boyd, J. E. and McCarthy, T. G. (1976). Cervical diameter after suction termination. *Br. Med. J.*, **1**, 68

4
Pre-evacuation cervical dilatation in termination of pregnancy

P. C. HO, S. T. LIANG, G. W. K. TANG
and H. K. MA

INTRODUCTION

Vacuum aspiration is the most common method of termination of pregnancy in the first trimester. Mechanical dilatation of the cervix can lead to cervical laceration and uterine perforation. There is also concern about the effect of cervical injury on subsequent reproductive performance[1,2]. Therefore various types of natural prostaglandins and prostaglandin analogues have been used to dilate the cervix before vacuum aspiration in order to reduce the incidence of trauma to the cervix. Although most of the studies reported were not properly controlled, the data from the few controlled trials did show that some natural prostaglandins and prostaglandin analogues were effective in pre-evacuation cervical dilatation[3-6]. It is interesting that a significant proportion of primigravid patients (11%) treated with placebo pessaries had a cervical dilatation of 8 mm or more[6]. This may be due to the release of endogenous prostaglandins during vaginal insertion[7] or it may just be the result of cervical changes during pregnancy. So far the possible effects of placebo vaginal pessaries have not been studied.

16,16-dimethyl-*trans*-Δ^2 PGE$_1$ methyl ester (ONO-802) is a new stable prostaglandin analogue. Given vaginally in repeated doses, it is effective in inducing abortion in the first trimester of pregnancy[8,9].

43

There is also suggestive evidence that a single dose of ONO-802 vaginal pessary 3 hours before vacuum aspiration is effective in dilating the cervix with minimal side-effects[10]. Therefore we have conducted a double-blind placebo-controlled trial in the Department of Obstetrics and Gynaecology, University of Hong Kong. The aims are to find out: (1) the cervical dilatation in the first trimester of pregnancy, (2) the influence of insertion of placebo pessaries and (3) the efficacy of ONO-802 1 mg vaginal pessaries in preoperative cervical dilatation prior to vacuum aspiration for termination of first trimester pregnancy.

PATIENTS AND METHODS

Both primigravidae and multigravidae admitted into the University Gynaecological Unit, Queen Mary Hospital and Tsan Yuk Hospital for termination of first trimester pregnancy were studied. Patients who showed signs or symptoms of spontaneous abortion, past history of atopic diseases or any serious medical complications were excluded.

In the first part of the study, the cervical dilatation in patients not receiving any form of treatment was studied. After induction of general anaesthesia, the cervical dilatation was measured by passing the Hegar dilators in descending order and the diameter of the largest dilator that could be passed without resistance was noted.

The second part of the study was a double-blind placebo-controlled trial. One hundred and twenty pessaries sequentially numbered were supplied by the Ono Pharmaceutical Company. The numbering sequence was determined from a randomization schedule constructed to include five ONO-802 1 mg pessaries and five placebo pessaries in random order in each consecutive group of ten pessaries. Pessaries numbered 1–70 were allocated to multigravid patients and 71–120 were allocated to primigravid patients. The randomization code was not broken until the completion of the study.

Three hours before vacuum aspiration, one pessary was inserted into the posterior fornix of the patient's vagina. The blood pressure, pulse and temperature were recorded hourly and the side-effects were noted. All the vacuum aspirations were done under general anaesthesia and the cervical dilatation was measured as described above. If necessary, further dilatation to the size appropriate for the gestational age was carried out and vacuum aspiration was performed with a plastic Karman catheter. Blood loss during vacuum aspiration was estimated by measuring the volume of blood in the jar including the products of conception. Any complication during and after the operation was noted. The patient was asked to return for follow-up 4 weeks after the operation.

RESULTS

Altogether 70 primigravid and 125 multigravid patients were studied. The clinical characteristics of the patients are shown in Table 4.1. There is no significant difference in mean age and gestational age among the three groups of patients. The details of the cervical state at the time of vacuum aspiration are show in Table 4.2. In both primigravid and multigravid patients, the number of patients in the ONO-802 group with cervical dilatation of 8 mm or more is significantly higher than that in the no-treatment group and the placebo group ($p < 0.01$ by the Chi-square test). The difference between the no-treatment group and the placebo group is not statistically significant.

Table 4.1   Characteristics of patients

	No treatment	Placebo	ONO-802
Primigravida			
Number	24	23	23
Mean age in years (SD)	21.5 (4.5)	21.1 (3.7)	21.2 (3.2)
Mean gestational age in weeks (SD)	9.6 (1.3)	9.7 (1.7)	10.0 (1.4)
Multigravida			
Number	60	30	35
Mean age in years (SD)	33.7 (6.6)	33.3 (5.1)	33.1 (5.3)
Mean gestational age in weeks (SD)	9.1 (1.2)	9.8 (1.2)	10.3 (1.3)

SD = standard deviation

Table 4.2   Details of cervical state at the time of vacuum aspiration

	No treatment	Placebo	ONO-802
Primigravida			
Mean cervical dilatation in mm (SD)	5.6 (1.6)	6.7 (1.4)	8.1 (1.7)
Cervical dilatation ⩾8 mm (%)	3 (13%)	6 (26%)	14 (61%)
Further dilatation not necessary (%)	NA	1 (4%)	9 (39%)
Multigravida			
Mean cervical dilatation in mm (SD)	6.5 (1.8)	6.8 (1.7)	8.8 (2.2)
Cervical dilatation ⩾8 mm (%)	14 (23%)	9 (30%)	26 (74%)
Further dilatation not necessary (%)	NA	4 (13%)	13 (37%)

NA = not available

Table 4.3 Blood loss and operative complications

	Placebo	ONO-802
Primigravida		
Blood loss in ml (SD)	157.8 (131.3)	112.0 (68.1)
Blood loss ≥ 200 ml (%)	10 (43%)	1 (4%)
Operative complications	1*	0
Multigravida		
Blood loss in ml (SD)	156.0 (115.0)	83.3 (40.7)
Blood loss ≥ 200 ml (%)	10 (33.3%)	0 (0%)
Operative complications	0	0

*Cervical laceration

The number of patients in the ONO-802 group not requiring further cervical dilatation is also significantly higher than that in the placebo group ($p < 0.02$ in primigravidae and $p < 0.05$ in multigravidae by the Chi-square test).

The blood loss at operation and operative complications are shown in Table 4.3. For both primigravidae and multigravidae, the number of patients in the ONO-802 group with blood loss of 200 ml or more is significantly less than that in the placebo group ($p < 0.01$ by the Chi-square test). One patient in the placebo group sustained a cervical laceration during operation.

The side-effects before operation are shown in Table 4.4. Only 10.3% of the patients had one or two episodes of vomiting and the average number of episodes of vomiting per patient is 0.14. Diarrhoea occurred in 1.7% of patients and the average number of episodes of diarrhoea per patient is 0.04. Transient pyrexia occurred in 8.6% of patients. None of the patients had uterine pain severe enough to require analgesics.

Forty-nine patients (84.5%) in the ONO-802 group and 40 patients (75.5%) in the placebo group returned for follow-up. The significant complications that developed after discharge from hospital are shown in Table 4.5.

Table 4.4 Incidence of side-effects

	Placebo	ONO-802
Vomiting	1 (1.9%)	6 (10.3%)
Diarrhoea	0 (0%)	1 (1.7%)
Transient pyrexia (> 37.5 °C)	1 (1.9%)	5 (8.6%)

Table 4.5 Complications after discharge from hospital

	Placebo	ONO-802
Incomplete abortion	0	1
Abdominal pain	2	1
Dysfunctional uterine bleeding	1	1
Pelvic infection	1	0

DISCUSSION

An ideal method of pre-evacuation cervical dilatation should be simple and easy to use, effective within a short time, free from side-effects, economical and acceptable to the patients. Although many methods have been reported, most of the studies have been uncontrolled trials and comparative trials are relatively few. Therefore there is as yet no general consensus as to the best method of pre-evacuation cervical dilatation.

The use of laminaria tents and Nelaton catheters has been claimed to be effective and practical method of pre-evacuation cervical dilatation[11, 12]. To be fully effective, however, a long insertion–evacuation interval of 12 hours is necessary. They need to be inserted through the internal cervical os and trained medical staff are required for proper insertion. Complications such as creation of false passages, difficulty in removing laminaria tents, extrauterine displacement have also been reported.

The results of trials with natural prostaglandins are disappointing. Low doses of PGE_2 and $PGF_{2\alpha}$ are ineffective vaginally[6, 13]. Higher doses are more effective but are associated with gastro-intestinal side-effects in 30–40% of patients[3, 6].

The use of prostaglandin analogues given by the extra-amniotic and intracervical routes is effective in pre-evacuation cervical dilatation[4, 14] but again trained medical staff are required for proper administration.

Recently three stable prostaglandin E analogues have become available for clinical trials: ONO-802, 16-phenoxy-ω-17,18,19,20-tetranor PGE_2 methylsulfonylamide (Sulprostone) and 9-deoxo-16,16-dimethyl-9-methylene prostaglandin E_2. They appear to be effective in dilating the cervix within 3 hours of administration[10, 15]. Sulprostone can be given intramuscularly and the other two analogues vaginally. Side-effects have been minimal.

Our study is a double-blind placebo-controlled trial and the factors of selection bias and observer bias are eliminated. Our results show that the insertion of placebo pessaries did not influence the cervical state, but the ONO-802 1 mg pessaries inserted vaginally 3 hours before operation produced significant cervical dilatation so that further mechanical dilatation was not necessary in 39% of primigravidae and 37% of multigravidae. The blood loss was also significantly reduced by pre-evacuation treatment with ONO-802 pessaries. This regime of pre-evacuation cervical dilatation is simple and easy. Since it is effective even with a short insertion–evacuation interval of 3 hours, it can be incorporated into an outpatient abortion service. Moreover the side-effects are mild and infrequent. Therefore it can be considered as one of the useful methods for pre-evacuation cervical dilatation.

References

1 Wright, C. S. W., Campbell, S. and Beazley, J. (1972). Second trimester abortion after vaginal termination of pregnancy. *Lancet*, **1**, 1278
2 Pantelakis, S. N., Papadimitriou, G. C. and Doxiadis, S. A. (1973). Influence of induced and spontaneous abortions on the outcome of subsequent pregnancies. *Am. J. Obstet. Gynaecol*, **116**, 799
3 Brenner, W. E., Dingfelder, J. R., Staurovsky, L. G. and Hendricks, C. H. (1973). Vaginally administered $PGF_{2\alpha}$ for cervical dilatation in nulliparas prior to suction curettage. *Prostaglandins*, **4**, 819
4 Cheng, M. C. E., Karim, S. M. M. and Ratnam, S. S. (1975). Pre-operative cervical dilatation with 15(S)-15-methyl prostaglandin E_2 methyl ester in first trimester nulliparae – a double blind study. *Contraception*, **12**, 59
5 WHO Prostaglandin Task Force (1981). Vaginal administration of 15-methyl $PGF_{2\alpha}$ methyl ester for pre-operative cervical dilatation. *Contraception*, **23**, 251
6 Mackenzie, I. Z. and Fry, A. (1981). Prostaglandin E_2 pessaries to facilitate first trimester aspiration termination. *Br. J. Obstet. Gynaecol.*, **88**, 1033
7 Mitchell, M. D., Flint, A. P. F., Bibby, J., Brunt, J., Arnold, J. M., Anderson, A. B. M. and Turnbull, A. C. (1977). Rapid increases in plasma prostaglandin concentrations after vaginal examination and amniotomy. *Br. Med. J.*, **2**, 1183
8 Nakano, R., Hata, H., Sasaki, K. and Yamamoto, M. (1980). The use of prostaglandin E_1 analogue pessaries in patients having first trimester induced abortions. *Br. J. Obstet. Gynaecol.*, **87**, 287
9 Smith, S. K. and Baird, D. T. (1980). The use of 16,16-dimethyl-*trans*-Δ^2 PGE_1 methyl ester (ONO-802) vaginal suppositories for termination of early pregnancy. A comparative study. *Br. J. Obstet. Gynaecol.*, **87**, 712
10 Prasad, R. N. V., Lim, C., Wong, Y. C., Karim, S. M. M. and Ratnam, S. S. (1978). Vaginal administration of 16,16-dimethyl-*trans*-Δ^2 PGE_1 methyl ester (ONO-802) for pre-operative cervical dilatation in first trimester nulliparous pregnancy. *Singapore J. Obstet. Gynaecol.*, **9**, 69
11 Hale, R. W. and Pion, R. J. (1972). Laminaria: an underutilized clinical adjunct. *Clin. Obstet Gynaecol.*, **15**, 829
12 Manabe, Y. and Manabe, A. (1981). Nelaton catheter versus laminaria for a safe and gradual cervical dilatation. *Contraception*, **24**, 53
13 Quinn, M. A., Jalland, M., Wein, R. and Kloss, M. (1981). Vaginal prostaglandin $F_{2\alpha}$ gel before first trimester terminaton of pregnancy. *Aust. N.Z. J. Obstet. Gynaecol.*, **21**, 93

14 Karim, S. M. M., Ratnam, S. S., Selvadurai, V., Wun, W. and Prasad, R. N. V. (1977). Cervical dilatation with 16,6-dimethyl PGE_2 p-benzaldehyde semicarbazone ester prior to vacuum aspiration in first trimester nulliparae. *Prostaglandins*, **13**, 333

15 Bygdeman, M., Bremme, K., Christensen, N., Lundström, V. and Gréen, K. (1980). A comparison of two stable prostaglandin E analogues for termination of early pregnancy and for cervical dilatation. *Contraception*, **22**, 471

5
Cervagem clinical trials review. Part I: Pre-operative cervical dilatation in pregnant women

S. A. PITTS

A lot has been written in recent years about the potential hazards of forceful dilatation of the cervix. The case implicating cervical lacerations, resulting from such mechanical dilatation, with cervical incompetence, mid-trimester abortion and premature delivery in subsequent pregnancies is still not yet proven. However, there is undoubtedly sufficient concern amongst clinicians to have warranted research into methods of reducing both overt and latent cervical damage at operation.

Sultan Karim started our work in cervical dilatation – a dose ranging study of 0.1, 0.5, 1.0 and 1.5 mg of ONO-802 given 3 h prior to evacuation of the uterus[1] (Table 5.1). From these results the 1.0 mg dosage was chosen for future evaluation. In 1978, Prasad[2] and his co-workers confirmed the efficacy of this dose in a study of 90 nulliparous patients. They found that in 80% of the patients, a cervical dilatation of 8 mm or greater was achieved, and that in these patients no further dilatation was necessary to perform the operation. In the remaining 20% of patients a dilatation of 5–7 mm, associated with cervical softening, allowed easy further dilatation up to size necessary to effect the procedure (Table 5.2). In both this study and Karim's dose-ranging study, the only side-effect reported was mild uterine cramp.

Table 5.1   Cervical dilatation obtained with a single dose of Cervagem 3 hours pre-opertively

Cervical dilatation	Dose of Cervagem (vaginal)			
	0.1 mg	0.5 mg	1.0 mg	1.5 mg
	No. of patients	No. of patients	No. of patients	No. of patients
3 mm or less	10	0	0	0
4 mm	4	0	0	0
5 mm	5	1	0	0
6 mm	1	5	2	0
7 mm	0	5	4	2
8 mm	0	6	15	8
9 mm	0	2	14	5
10 mm	0	1	4	3
11 mm	0	0	1	2
Total	20	20	40	20

Source: Karim (1977)[1]

Table 5.2   Efficacy of a single Cervagem 1 mg vaginal pessary

Cervical dilatation (mm)	Cervical dilatation 3 h after Cervagem administration		
	No. of patients	Total	%
5	3 ⎫		
6	6 ⎬	18	20
7	9 ⎭		
8	28 ⎫		
9	26 ⎪		
10	13 ⎬	72	80
11	5 ⎭		

Source: Prasad et al. (1979)[2]

More recently Welch and Elder conducted a study in 43 primigravid women who had had no previous transcervical operations[3]. Their results showed a significant degree of pre-operative cervical dilatation in those patients who received a Cervagem 1 mg pessary approximately 3 h prior to the operation (Table 5.3). They also found that the force required to insert the maximum size of dilator necessary was significantly reduced when compared to a control group who received no

Table 5.3 Cervical dilatation in treatment (Cervagem 1 mg) and control (no pre-treatment) groups

	Cervagem group (n = 25)	Control group (n = 18)	Significance level
Maximum diameter (mm) of dilator inserted with unrecordable pressure of <0.3 kg	6.36 ±2.8	4.06 ±2.42	$p < 0.001$
Force required to insert maximum size of dilator (kg)	0.86 ±0.31	1.16 ±0.17	$p < 0.001$
Diameter of maximum size of dilator used (mm)	9.44 ±1.91	8.98 ±2.13	NS

Values are mean ±1 SD
Source: Welch and Elder (1982)[3]

pre-treatment. To show that the groups were comparable, the authors recorded the size of the maximum dilator that was used to effect the procedure (Table 5.3). In this study, 44% of patients experienced mild to moderate pre-operative pain, three patients were nauseated, one vomited but none of the patients required any treatment for these symptoms.

In 1981, a six-centre study was set up in Scandinavia. Three centres have completed their part of the trial and the data were presented as an abstract[4] at the Florence Conference in May 1982. I would like to take this opportunity on behalf of Drs. Kajanoja, Mandelin, Ylikorkala and Mäkilä to present a more detailed analysis of these results.

This was a double-blind placebo-controlled multicentre trial, basically of the same design as that conducted by Professor Ma's group (see Chapter 4, Dr Ho's presentation). Each centre admitted 60 nulliparous patients. For the purpose of this study, nulliparous was defined as patients in their first pregnancy or where previous pregnancies had ended before completing the 12th week. Patients were excluded if they showed signs or symptoms of spontaneous abortion or if they had a serious medical disorder. All patients were admitted according to the local legal requirements for first trimester termination of pregnancy under general anaesthetic.

A break-down of the patients who were admitted to these three centres is presented in Table 5.4. In terms of their general characteristics, the two groups are very comparable (Table 5.5). Gestational

Table 5.4 Multicentre study of cervical dilatation with Cervagem 1 mg vaginal pessary

Patients admitted to the first 3 centres		
	Cervagem group	*Placebo group*
Number entered	90	90
Number withdrawn	6	3
Total analysed	84	87
Follow-up losses	2	4
Reasons for withdrawals		
Multigravidae	4	1
Cervical os open prior to treatment	2	1
Pre-operative vaginal bleeding after treatment	0	1

Table 5.5 Multicentre study, patient details

	Cervagem group (n = 84)	*Placebo group* (n = 87)
Age (years)	22.4 ± 5.9	21.8 ± 4.5
Height (cm)	164.8 ± 5.2	164.5 ± 5.8
Weight (kg)	57.8 ± 9.0	57.7 ± 8.1
Gestational age (weeks & days)	9 wk 1 d ± 1 wk 2 d	8 wk 5 d ± 1 wk 1 d

Values are mean ± 1 SD

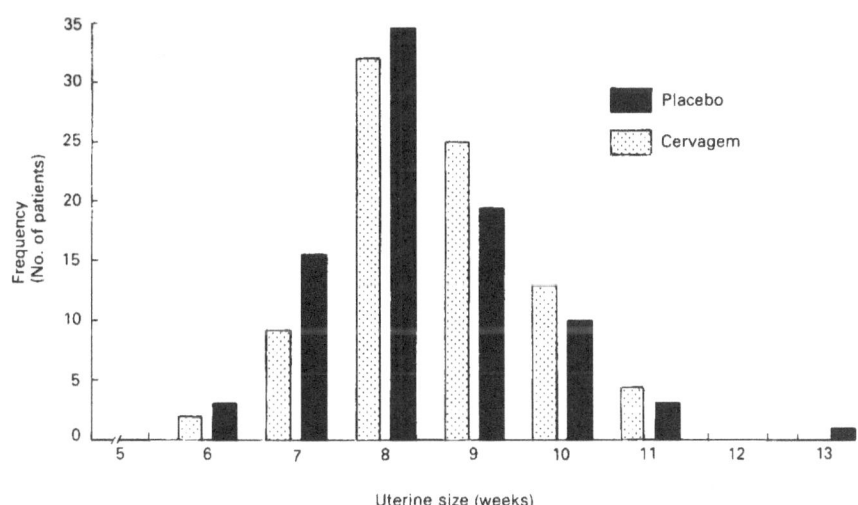

Figure 5.1 Multicentre study. Distribution of uterine size

age, calculated from the first day of the last menstrual period, correlated well with clinicians' assessment of the uterine size (Figure 5.1). (The patient with 13-week uterine size was a twin pregnancy of 11 weeks' gestation confirmed by ultrasound examination.) All of the patients in the study received a vaginal pessary approximately 3 h prior to the operation – the mean time in both groups was approximately 3 h 25 min, and the range was between 2½ and 6 h. The placebo and Cervagem pessaries were matched and therefore administration was observer and patient blind.

Side-effects and symptoms were recorded in the interval between the administration of the pessary and surgery, and are shown in Table 5.6.

Table 5.6   Multicentre study, pre-operative side-effects and symptoms

Side-effect/symptom	Cervagem group No. of patients	%	Placebo group No. of patients	%
None	38	45.2	58	66.7
Uterine pain				
Mild	26	31.0	21	24.1
Moderate	5	6.0	0	—
Severe	1	1.2	0	—
Vomiting	7	8.3	1	1.1
Nausea	2	2.4	1	1.1
Diarrhoea	2	2.4	0	—
Flushing	3	3.6	8	9.2
Backache	3	3.6	1	1.1
Headache	0	—	2	2.3
Others	1	1.2	5	5.7
Vaginal bleeding*	11	13.1	0	—

* Mean time to onset of vaginal bleeding 2 h 33 min ± 0 h 34 min

45% of patients in the Cervagem group experienced no side-effects at all compared with 67% in the placebo group. Flushing in both groups was not associated with any rise in temperature, and there were no noticeable effects on temperature, pulse or blood pressure in either group. No patients aborted prior to operation. At operation, the size of Hegar dilator which could be inserted without meeting resistance was recorded as the cervical dilatation achieved. The amount of pre-operative cervical dilatation in the Cervagem group had a median value of 7 mm and in the placebo group of 5 mm. As can be seen from

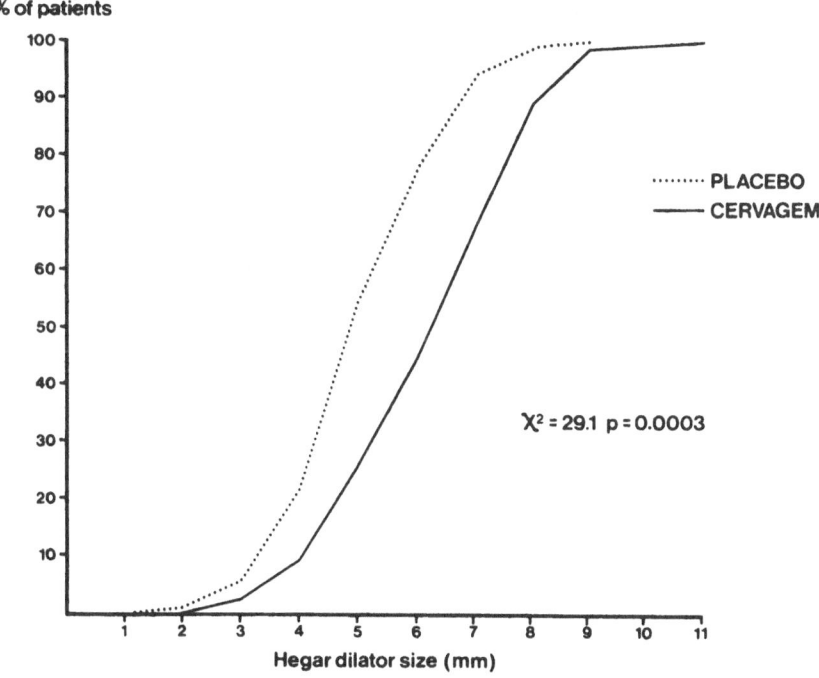

Figure 5.2   Multicentre study. Cumulative frequency graph of cervical dilatation prior to surgery

the cumulative frequency graph (Figure 5.2), there were two distinct populations and a Chi-square analysis shows them to be significantly different. Seventy-four per cent of the patients in the Cervagem group had a dilatation of 6 mm or greater (cf. 49% in the placebo group). Only eight patients (9%) in the Cervagem group had a dilatation of 4 mm or less (cf. 19 patients, or 22%, in the placebo group). One of these eight patients had significant cervical softening, and dilatation up to the size necessary to effect the procedure was considered easy.

We looked at factors which might be thought to affect the size of dilator that could be inserted without resistance. The obvious choice was the time elapsed between the administration of the pessary and surgery, however, with a time range of only 3½ h, we were unable to show any such effect. Where further dilatation was necessary, it was recorded as either easier, the same or more difficult than normal. The results are shown in Figure 5.3.

We have heard suggestions that there is reduction in operative blood loss in patients who receive pre-treatment with prostaglandins. Although there was a trend towards that in this series, none of the differences was significant (Table 5.7). The mean value for the Cervagem

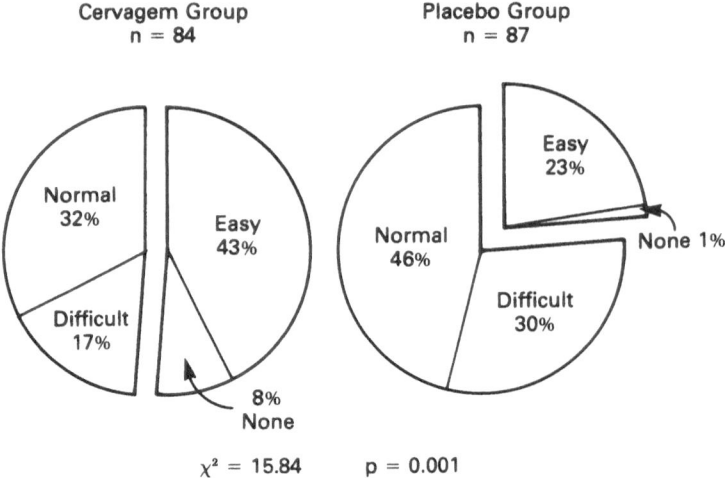

Figure 5.3   Multicentre study. Assessment of ease of mechanical dilatation

Table 5.7   Multicentre study, operative blood loss (ml)

	Mean	SD	Median	Mode
Cervagem group (n = 84)	96.1	47.4	90	150
Placebo group (n = 87)	112.9	74.4	110	150

None of the differences between placebo and Cervagem patients was statistically significant

group was lower than that for the placebo group and the standard deviation smaller. The median value was also lower than that of the placebo group but the mode (that value which was recorded most often) was the same in both treatment groups. The data in both groups were very skewed – only one patient in the Cervagem group had a blood loss greater than 150 ml. In the placebo group, there were two such patients, one who lost 400 ml and one who lost 550 ml. In both of these placebo group patients, dilatation was very difficult and the investigator attributed the high blood loss to this difficulty. As in Professor Ma's trial, the operative blood loss was estimated as the blood loss including the products of conception. We examined this in terms of gestational age but could find no correlation between the two variables.

Patients were observed for a minimum of 3 h post-operatively; no abnormalities or differences were recorded in temperature, pulse or blood pressure. There was no difference between the two groups in the recorded severity of post-operative bleeding. Haemoglobin estimations

Table 5.8 Multicentre study, post-operative side-effects and symptoms

Side-effect/symptom	Cervagem group No. of patients	%	Placebo group No. of patients	%
Uterine pain – Mild	23	27 ⎱	32	37 ⎱
– Moderate	20	24 ⎰ 57%	15	17 ⎰ 55%
– Severe	5	6 ⎰	1	1 ⎰
Analgesics given:	17	20 (35*)	13	15 (27*)
Vomiting	19	23	6	7
Antiemetics given:	6	7 (32†)	2	2 (33†)
Drowsiness	0	—	1	1

* % of patients experiencing pain who received analgesia
† % of patients experiencing vomiting who received antiemetics

made prior to treatment and immediately before discharge from hospital showed no difference either between the groups or in the pre- and post-operative values within the groups. Signs and symptoms recorded are shown in Table 5.8.

All but six patients returned for follow-up visit which was arranged between 2 and 4 weeks after the operation. The patients were asked about their duration of bleeding and asked to compare this loss with their usual menstrual loss. The duration of bleeding was the same in both groups (Table 5.9). When compared with their usual menstrual

Table 5.9 Multicentre study, duration of bleeding post-operatively

		Cervagem group (n = 82)	Placebo group (n = 82)	p value
Duration of bleeding (days)	mean	6.36	7.12	
	SD	±5.37	±5.54	0.38
	range	0 to 21	0 to 21	
Difference from duration	mean	1.26	2.18	
of usual menstrual	SD	±5.58	±5.44	0.28
flow (days)	range	– 6 to + 16	– 6 to + 16	

loss, the patients tended to bleed 1 or 2 days longer than they would normally do at menstruation. When the severity of post-operative bleeding was compared with usual menstruation, almost all the patients felt that their post-operative bleeding was less than their usual

Table 5.10 Multicentre study, severity of post-operative bleeding compared to usual menstruation

	Less than usual	*Same as usual*	*More than usual*
Cervagem group (n = 82)	76	5	1
Placebo group (n = 83)	75	7	1

menstruation, and only one patient in each group felt that her bleeding was more (Table 5.10).

Details of late post-operative complications were recorded at these follow-up visits and a total of 12 cases of endometritis were recorded – three in Cervagem-treated cases and nine in the placebo group; otherwise all patients were well. There were 29 intra-uterine contraceptive devices inserted at the operation, 13 in the Cervagem group and 16 in placebo group. 28 of these 29 were retained, the one loss occurring in a placebo-treated patient.

To conclude, we now have a body of evidence which seems amply to demonstrate the efficacy of Cervagem and to confirm the low incidence of side-effects. There have been no reported drug interactions.

References

1 Karim S. M. M. (1977). Data on file at May & Baker Ltd., Dagenham, Essex, UK
2 Prasad, R. N. V., Lim, C., Wong, Y. C., Karim, S. M. M. and Ratnam, S. S. (1978). Vaginal administration of 16,16-dimethyl-*trans*-Δ^2-PGE$_1$ methyl ester (ONO-802) for pre-operative cervical dilatation in first trimester nulliparous pregnancy. *Singapore J. Obstet. Gynaecol.*, **9**, 69
3 Welch, C. and Elder, M. G. (1982). Cervical dilatation with 16,16-dimethyl-*trans*-Δ^2-PGE$_1$ methyl ester vaginal pessaries before surgical termination of first trimester pregnancies. *Br. J. Obstet. Gynaecol.*, **89**, 849
4 Kajanoja, P., Mandelin, M., Mäkilä, U. M. and Ylikorkala, O. (1982). ONO-802 vaginal suppositories in pre-operative cervical softening. Presented at *Vth International Conference on Prostaglandins*, May 18–21 Florence, Italy (Abstract)

Discussion 2

(5) **Dr Choong Kuo Hsiang** (Malaysia): Your study would seem to confirm a lot of other studies that show that there is reduced bleeding with the use of ONO-802 prior to cervical dilatation. I would like to ask you how you account for this decrease in blood loss, how much of it is due to the decrease in cervical trauma, laceration etc. How much is it due to vasoconstrictor effect of PGs?

Dr Pack Chung Ho (Hong Kong): I don't think that cervical laceration is a significant factor in the blood loss because after all in our series only one patient had sustained a superficial cervical laceration. I think most of this (of course, I have no data to support) is probably related to the uterine contractions that are induced by ONO-802. This is my explanation. I wonder if Professor Karim has any explanation to offer.

Dr Karim: I would tend to agree with you because unlike other oxytocics (oxytocin, ergometrine), prostaglandins are able to stimulate the pregnant uterus in early pregnancy and this would be expected to reduce blood loss. Perhaps Professor Bygdeman would like to comment.

Dr Bygdeman: If you use laminaria tent for cervical dilatation, you could achieve approximately the same degree of cervical dilatation as with the PGs. In spite of this, the blood loss with PGs is less than with laminaria indicating that the contractions of the uterus are important for the blood loss.

(6) **Dr Khew Khoon Shin** (Singapore): The time spent on curettage in order to evacuate the uterus completely would vary from patient to patient and this may reflect in the blood loss. My question is, have you standardized both the placebo group and the PG-treated group as far as curettage is concerned?

Dr Pak Chung Ho: Well, we had this problem in mind and the blood loss may be related to the operator. This is the reason why we did the study in the form of a double-blind placebo-controlled trial. It is done at random. We do not know which is the placebo pessary and which is the PG-containing pessary. All the patients are managed in more or less a standard manner. We hope that in this way we have minimized the variables.

(7) **Dr Karim:** What is your procedure for evacuating the first trimester uterus? What size catheter do you use?

Dr Pak Chung Ho: It depends on the gestation and uterine size. Usually, for uterine size of about 8 weeks or less, we use an 8 mm plastic catheter, but for a uterus between 10 and 12 weeks, we tend to use a 10 mm catheter.

(8) **Dr Karim:** Dr Fylling, why did you choose $300\,\mu g$ Sulprostone?

Dr Fylling (Norway): We have some experience with Sulprostone, which we have used by different routes and different doses. We have a feeling that there is a dose somewhere between $300\,\mu g$ and $500\,\mu g$ which is effective and produces a lower incidence of side-effects.

(9) **Dr Karim:** If it was possible by repeated administration of either Cervagem or by intramuscular administration of Sulprostone to expel the fetus in the first trimester, say, with two or three dosages, would this have any advantage over using PGs only for cervical dilatation followed by vacuum aspiration?

Dr Fylling: My answer is 'no'.

(10) **Dr Fylling:** I have a few comments on all three papers including my own. From a clinical point, there may be a difference between nulliparous women and primigravidae. Secondly, it is difficult to estimate the degree of cervical dilatation precisely. We are missing an instrument that could objectively assess the degree of cervical dilatation. In the absence of such a method we have to accept some subjective variation. I hope somebody with technical knowhow can construct an instrument for us.

(11) **Dr Khew Khoon Shin:** Does Cervagem produce any pre-operative bleeding and was it measured?

Mrs Pitts (UK): Yes. There were 11 patients who bled pre-operatively with Cervagem in this series. The blood loss was not measured, but in most cases, it was noted down as spotting or less than 10 ml or was felt to be so slight as not worth reporting.

(12) **Dr Gibb** (Singapore): I have a couple of comments to make. Firstly, regarding method, it seems odd that multigravid patients should have been included. Secondly, the use of intrauterine contraceptive devices after termination is known to affect subsequent blood loss and perhaps they should not have been used in either group. Thirdly, Table 5.7, this suggests an abnormal distribution of results for blood loss or some defects in the sample. Is there some simple explanation for this which I have missed?

Mrs. Pitts: I said the distribution of blood loss was skewed and in one centre 150 ml of blood loss was recorded very often. In the other two centres, blood loss was generally towards the lower end of the scale. That is why the data are skewed and the medians tell you that 50% of the values have to be below 90 ml in the Cervagem group and below 110 ml in the placebo group. We looked at the data to see if there is any difference in patients who had IUCDs inserted in terms of post-operative blood loss, duration of bleeding and side-effects. These patients were evenly distributed between the groups. The data were analysed by multivariant analysis and nothing significant came out of it. With regard to the five multigravidae, one patient had had two previous Caesarean sections. There were two or three who had had hysterotomy terminations at about 16 weeks and one patient had had a termination at 14 weeks so they were protocol violations using our definition of the term 'nulliparous'.

(13) **Dr Teo Yu Keng** (Malaysia): In Table 5.6, you said there were 21 patients in the placebo group who experienced some pain. Can you explain how the pain comes about in the placebo group?

Mrs Pitts: No, I can't. But I am sure Dr Bygdeman or Dr Karim can.

Dr Bygdeman: I think the protocol used required that you inform the patient about the procedure, and the possible side-effects the treatment may cause, and that information includes information about uterine pain. That is the explanation. If you tell a patient that she should expect pain, even those treated with placebo will get it.

6
Clinical experience with selected prostaglandin analogues in obstetrics and gynaecology

M. BYGDEMAN, N. CHRISTENSEN
and K. GRÉEN

INTRODUCTION

The intra-uterine administration of naturally occurring prostaglandins, $PGF_{2\alpha}$ and PGE_2, has been in clinical use for termination of second trimester pregnancy for several years. More recently, different prostaglandin analogues have been developed offering the possibility of using non-invasive routes, e.g. vaginal or intramuscular. These analogues have been used not only for termination of second trimester pregnancy but also for dilatation of the cervical canal prior to vacuum aspiration and as a non-surgical alternative for termination of very early pregnancy.

This review will deal mainly with preoperative cervical dilatation, but the use of selected prostaglandin analogues administered by non-invasive routes for termination of early pregnancy and for termination of second trimester pregnancy will also be summarized briefly. The analogues to be discussed are 16,16-dimethyl-*trans*-Δ^2 PGE_1 methyl ester (16,16-dimethyl PGE_1), 9-deoxo-16,16-dimethyl-9-methylene PGE_2 (9-methylene PGE_2) (both administered vaginally), and 16-phenoxy-ω-17,18,19,20-tetranor PGE_2 methylsulfonylamide (16-phenoxy PGE_2) given as intramuscular injections. In contrast to previously available PGE analogues, these new analogues seem to be sufficiently stable for routine clinical use and the effective dose schedules seem to be associated with a significantly lower frequency of gastro-intestinal side-effects than analogues belonging to the PGF series. In the near future it is likely that these compounds will replace, partly or entirely, other non-surgical methods in current use for termination of normal and abnormal pregnancy. Comparative studies using all these analogues have not been published previously. The data presented in this review are mainly based on studies performed in our department[1-3].

TERMINATION OF EARLY PREGNANCY

Patients and methods

This comparative study included 253 healthy women with an apparently normal pregnancy (judged from plasma β-hCG and gynaecological examination) and amenorrhea of 49 days or less. After being informed, all patients accepted a non-surgical procedure for pregnancy termination.

The patients received one of three alternative treatments:

(1) Intramuscular injections of 16-phenoxy PGE_2, 0.5 mg three times at 3-hourly interval.

(2) Vaginal suppositories containing 1.0 mg 16,16-dimethyl PGE_1 five times at 3-hourly interval.

(3) Vaginal suppositories containing 9-methylene PGE_2, 75 mg followed by 30 mg 6 hours later or 60 mg plus 45 mg with the same time interval.

The majority of patients were treated in the hospital during the day but on an outpatient basis. However, among the patients receiving treatment schedule No. 3, a group of 100 women were selected who agreed to treat themselves at home. A prerequisite for treatment at home was at least one previous pregnancy.

All patients attended two follow-up visits, 1 and 2 weeks after the treatment. At the follow-up visits haemoglobin value and plasma β-hCG were measured and at the second visit a gynaecological examination was performed. At the second follow-up visit the outcome of therapy was preliminarily judged as complete abortion, incomplete abortion, or non-interrupted pregnancy. The judgement was based on the duration and amount of bleeding, plasma β-hCG, gynaecological examination, and, if it was not obvious that the patient had aborted completely, ultrasound examination. If curettage was found necessary during the time from the second follow-up visit to the first menstruation, the outcome of treatment was based on the histopathological examination.

Results and comments

As illustrated in Figure 6.1, all the three PGE analogues were highly effective in terminating early pregnancy. The frequency of complete

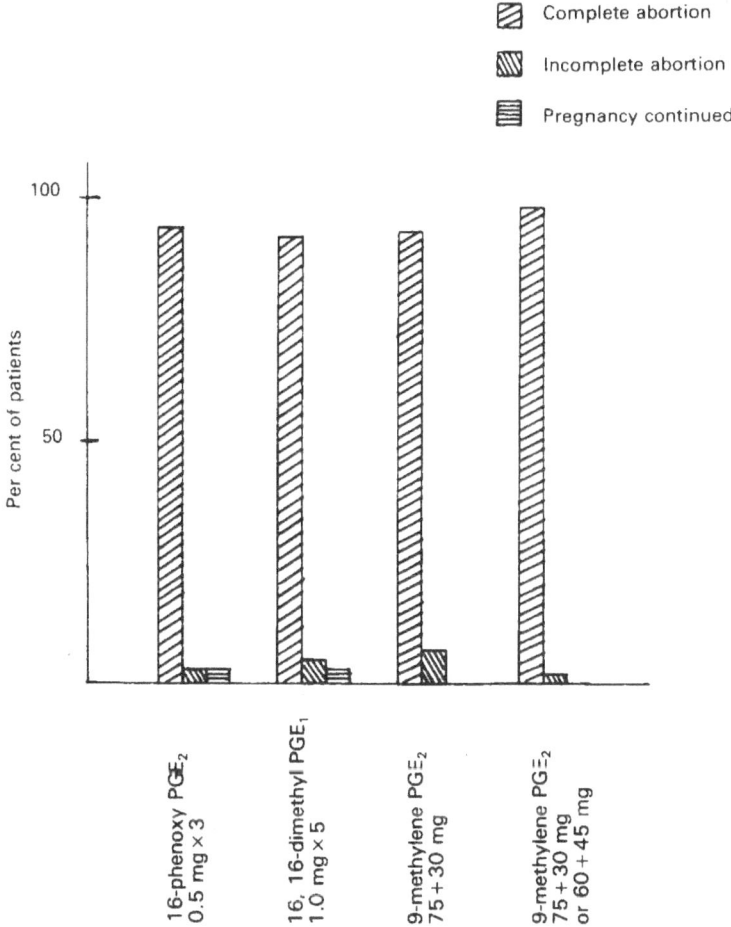

Figure 6.1 Termination of very early pregnancy by different prostaglandin analogues. The first three groups were treated in the hospital on an outpatient basis. In the fourth group the patients treated themselves at home

abortion varied between 92% and 94% for the three different treatment schedules. The success rate was even higher (96%) in the group of patients treated at home with 9-methylene PGE_2. The frequency of complete abortion (92–96%) is comparable with that reported previously for PGF analogues and also similar to that found for vacuum aspiration with the Karman catheter during the same period of gestation[4,5].

In rare cases the treatment may fail. To avoid continuation of pregnancy in these patients, a 100% follow-up is necessary. However, it must be pointed out that a similar risk for failed treatment also

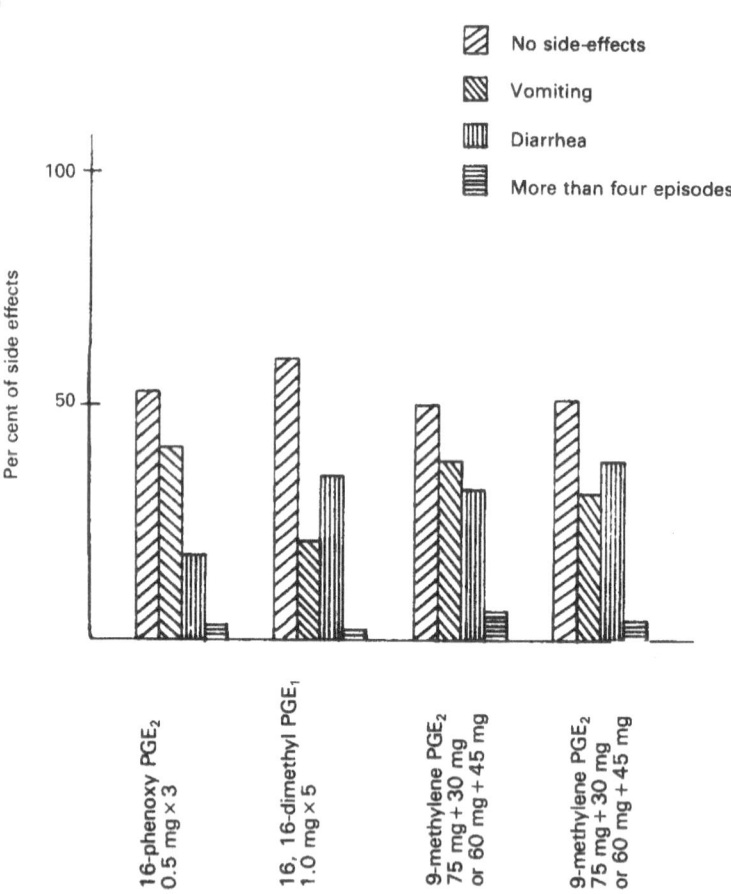

Figure 6.2 Gastro-intestinal side-effects following termination of very early pregnancy by different prostaglandin analogues. The first three groups were treated in the hospital on an outpatient basis. In the fourth group the patients treated themselves at home

applies to vacuum aspiration if performed during the same period of gestation.

The frequency of gastro-intestinal side-effects was also very similar for the three E analogues (Figure 6.2). Between 50 and 60% of the patients experienced no vomiting or diarrhoea. The percentage of patients with more than four episodes of both symptoms together was 6% or less, which is a much lower frequency than that reported earlier for vaginal administration of classical prostaglandins and analogues of the PGF series[6].

The only difference between the three compounds in the present study was the need for analgesic injections and the degree of temperature elevation. Patients treated with 16-phenoxy PGE$_2$ needed analgesic injections more often than patients treated with either 16,16-dimethyl PGE$_1$ or 9-methylene PGE$_2$. One reason for this difference could be the route of administration. Following intramuscular administration the compound is more rapidly absorbed than following vaginal administration, resulting in a more pronounced elevation of the intra-uterine pressure. However, the most obvious difference was between hospital and home treated patients. Only 2% of the latter group of patients experienced severe uterine pain. On the other hand, temperature elevation was more common if 9-methylene PGE$_2$ was used, but did not exceed 40 °C with the dose schedule used. During treatment or during the subsequent days none of the patients experienced heavy bleeding necessitating intervention. The mean amount of blood loss during the entire bleeding period was 61.7 ml (range 21–150 ml). The only patients in whom bleeding could cause problems were those with an incomplete abortion often associated with a prolonged but not heavy bleeding. No patient was readmitted to the hospital because of pelvic inflammatory disease. However, 0–2% of the patients in the different treatment groups received antibiotic treatment on an ambulatory basis.

The results of the present study confirm our previous report[6], i.e. the amount of bleeding and the frequency of pelvic inflammatory disease is rarely a problem in prostaglandin-induced early abortion, at least if the treatment is restricted to the first 3 weeks following a missed menstrual period.

Conclusions

It may be concluded that the new prostaglandin E analogues now available for clinical trials are highly effective in terminating early pregnancy and are superior to previously used PGF analogues with regard to side-effects, even if administered by non-invasive routes. The efficacy and safety of the treatment seems good enough to allow self-treatment at home. In the first study in which this possibility was evaluated the efficacy and acceptability was good, at least in well-informed patients. It may now be appropriate to initiate studies which randomly compare vacuum aspiration with the non-surgical procedures.

PREOPERATIVE CERVICAL DILATATION

Patients and methods

This comparative study included 550 patients in the 8th–12th week of pregnancy, admitted to the hospital for termination of pregnancy. The patients received one of the following treatments: either 0.5 mg or 1.0 mg 15-methyl $PGF_{2\alpha}$ methyl ester for 3 h, 1.0 mg 16,16-dimethyl-*trans*-Δ^2 PGE_1 methyl ester for 3, 6 or 12 h, 0.25 mg 16-phenoxy-ω-17,18,19,20-tetranor PGE_2 methylsulfonylamide for 3 h, or 0.5 mg of the same compound for 3 and 12 h or one medium-size laminaria tent for 3 h. The prostaglandin analogues were administered as vaginal suppositories with the exception of 16-phenoxy-ω-17,18,19,20-tetranor PGE_2 methylsulfonylamide, which was given as intramuscular injections. The patients in the different treatment groups were comparable with regard to mean age (25.6 years; range 24.2–26.3), duration of pregnancy (10.7 weeks; range 10–11), and percentage of nulliparous women (91.5%; range 80–97).

The surgical procedure was the same in all patients. The patients were operated on with paracervical block after preoperative sedation. The degree of cervical dilatation was measured by the size of the largest Hegar dilator that could be inserted through the cervical canal without resistance. Operative bleeding was measured after sieving the products of conceptus. Two doctors, both experienced with the procedure, alternated in performing the vacuum aspirations.

Duration of pregnancy was estimated based on the duration of amenorrhoea and uterine size. If these two measurements disagreed, ultrasound examination was performed.

The patients were carefully supervised during the treatment period and for at least 3 hours following the vacuum aspiration, for bleeding, side-effects, demand for analgesic injections, preoperative abortions, etc.

Results and comments

The degree of cervical dilatation was related to the duration of prostaglandin treatment. For the three E analogues the mean cervical dilatation after the 3-hour pretreatment was between 6.9 and 7.9 mm. It increased to 8.6–9.1 mm after 6 h of pretreatment and to 9.3–10.0 mm if the treatment period was extended to 12 h.

The frequency of abortion prior to the scheduled time for vacuum aspiration, the need for analgesic injections, and gastro-intestinal side-effects also significantly increased with time.

In Figure 6.3 is illustrated the increase in both efficacy and side-effects in relation to the duration of treatment following vaginal administration of 1.0 mg 16,16-dimethyl-*trans*-Δ^2 PGE$_1$ methyl ester.

The outcome of therapy with all the prostaglandin analogues was compared after a 3-hour observation period (Table 6.1). 1.0 mg of 15-methyl PGF$_{2\alpha}$ methyl ester, 0.5 mg of 16-phenoxy-ω-17,18,19,20-tetranor PGE$_2$ methylsulfonylamide, 30 mg of 9-deoxo-16,16-dimethyl-9-methylene PGE$_2$, and 1.0 mg of 16,16-dimethyl-*trans*-Δ^2 PGE$_1$ methyl ester all resulted in a mean cervical dilatation of 7.2–7.9 mm if the

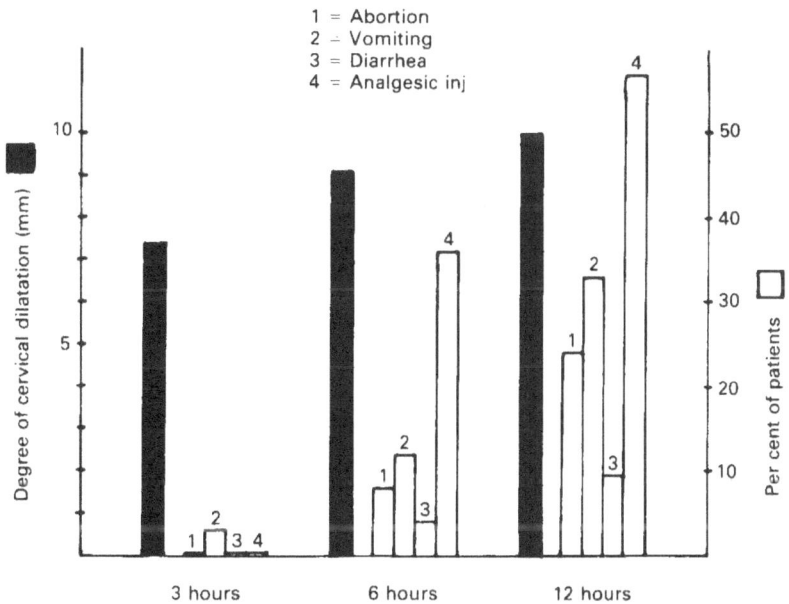

Figure 6.3   Preoperative cervical dilatation in late first trimester patients by vaginal administration of 1.0 mg of 16,16-dimethyl-*trans*-Δ^2 PGE$_1$ methyl ester. Vacuum aspiration was performed 3, 6 or 12 h after the start of therapy

Table 6.1 **Degree of cervical dilatation following a 3-hour pretreatment period with different prostaglandin analogues and one medium size laminaria tent**

Compound	Dose (mg)	Mean cervical dilatation ($\pm SD$) (mm)	Patients with a dilatation of 7 mm or more (%)
15-methyl PGF$_{2\alpha}$ methyl ester	0.5	6.5 ± 1.6	47†
15-methyl PGF$_{2\alpha}$ methyl ester	1.0	7.2 ± 1.5	63†
16,16-dimethyl-*trans*-Δ^2 PGE$_1$ methyl ester	1.0	7.4 ± 2.1*	59†
9-deoxo-16,16-dimethyl-9-methylene-PGE$_2$	30	7.9 ± 1.7*	85†
16-phenoxy-ω-17,18,19,20-tetranor PGE$_2$ methyl sulfonylamide	0.25	6.9 ± 1.8	59†
16-phenoxy-ω-17,18,19,20-tetranor PGE$_2$ methyl sulfonylamide	0.5	7.4 ± 1.6*	75†
One laminaria tent, medium size		6.1 ± 0.7	20

* Significantly different from laminaria ($p < 0.05$; contrasts based on one-way analysis of variance)

† Significantly different from laminaria ($p < 0.05$; χ^2)

pretreatment period was 3 h. No statistically significant differences were found for these treatment schedules if calculated on the degree of cervical dilatation or on the number of patients with a cervical dilatation of 7 mm or more.

With all prostaglandin treatment schedules, the number of patients with a cervical dilatation of 7 mm or more was significantly higher than following pretreatment with one medium-size laminaria tent ($p < 0.05$–0.001).

The frequency of gastro-intestinal side-effects (vomiting and/or diarrhoea) was low for all the prostaglandin treatments if the pretreatment period was 3 h. With all dose schedules except 0.5 mg of 16-phenoxy PGE$_2$ methylsulfonylamide and 1.0 mg of 15-methyl PGF$_{2\alpha}$ methyl ester, gastro-intestinal side-effects occurred in 7% or less of the patients and were not statistically significantly different from those for laminaria tent.

If different prostaglandin analogues are to be compared with regard to the frequency of side-effects, it is important that equivalent dose schedules are used, i.e. a dose resulting in the same degree of cervical dilatation. With this prerequisite in mind, 1.0 mg of 16,16-dimethyl-*trans*-Δ^2 PGE$_1$ methyl ester and 30 mg of 9-deoxo-16,16-dimethyl-9-methylene PGE$_2$ were preferable to 1.0 mg of 15-methyl PGF$_{2\alpha}$ methyl ester and to 0.5 mg of 16-phenoxy-ω-17,18,19,20-tetranor PGE$_2$ methyl sulfonylamide if the pretreatment period was 3 h. The higher frequency of vomiting and diarrhoea following 16-phenoxy-ω-17,18,19,20-tetranor PGE$_2$ methyl sulfonylamide is most likely due to the mode of administration. Following intramuscular injection the compound is more rapidly absorbed into the circulation than following vaginal administration. That the frequency of gastro-intestinal side-effects was the same for 16-phenoxy-ω-17,18,19,20-tetranor PGE$_2$ methyl sulfonyl-amide as for the other E analogues if the treatment period was extended to 12 hours supports this assumption. If the vaginal route is used the compound is also washed out from the vagina at vacuum aspiration. The higher frequency of gastro-intestinal side-effects following vaginal administration of the PGF analogue is most likely due to the fact that these analogues in general discriminate less effectively between uterine and gastro-intestinal smooth muscle. Temperature elevation is sometimes a problem following treatment with PGE analogues. With the low doses used in the present study this was rarely observed and in no case disturbing for the patient.

From the present and previous studies[7] it is clear that a pretreatment period of 12 h is preferable if a maximum dilatation of the cervical canal is aimed at. However, a 3-hour pretreatment period is sufficient in many patients and in the majority of the remaining ones additional mechanical dilatation is an easy procedure. The low frequency of gastro-intestinal side-effects and pain and the fact that the procedure allows for outpatient care makes the 3-hour pretreatment period the preferable one. A short pretreatment also eliminates the risk of abortion prior to the scheduled time of vacuum aspiration.

The percentage of patients with blood loss of 50 ml or more was significantly higher following treatment with laminaria than following treatment with PGE analogues (Table 6.2). It is well known that increased uterine contractility may reduce the blood loss during vacuum aspiration. It is likely that prostaglandin treatment stimulates uterine contractility more effectively than laminaria tent. The increased con-tractility may facilitate the surgical removal of the conceptus due to a partial separation of the placenta prior to surgery and because the uterine wall is easily recognized.

Conclusions

It is generally agreed that the frequency of complications following vacuum aspiration or dilatation and curettage (D & C) increases with increasing gestational age[8]. Some of these complications, i.e. cervical injury and uterine perforation, are directly related to the mechanical dilatation necessary for the procedure, especially during the latter part of the first trimester and the early part of the second trimester. Other complications, e.g. haemorrhage and incomplete evacuation of the conceptus, may possibly be related to an insufficient or difficult dilatation. In a previous multicentre study it was shown that treatment with 1.0 mg of 15-methyl $PGF_{2\alpha}$ methyl ester during 3 or 12 hours

Table 6.2 Comparison of different prostaglandin analogues and laminaria for preoperative dilatation of the cervix in late first trimester abortion. Amount of blood loss at vacuum aspiration

Compound	No. of patients	Dose (mg)	Mean blood loss (ml)	Patients with a blood loss of more than 50 ml (%)
15-methyl $PGF_{2\alpha}$ methyl ester	80	0.5	44	46
15-methyl $PGF_{2\alpha}$ methyl ester	75	1.0	39	35
16,16-dimethyl-trans-Δ^2 PGE_1 methyl ester	34	1.0	20	6*
9-deoxo-16,16-dimethyl-9-methylene PGE_2	27	30	28	11*
16-phenoxy-ω-17,18,19,20-tetranor PGE_2 methylsulfonylamide	100	0.25	31	21*
16-phenoxy-ω-17,18,19,20-tetranor PGE_2 methylsulfonylamide	39	0.5	34	25*
One laminaria tent, medium size	30		59	53*

* Significantly different from laminaria ($p < 0.05$; χ^2)

prior to vacuum aspiration in primigravid patients in comparison with placebo resulted in a significant dilatation of the cervical canal and a reduction in the frequency of operative and post-operative complications. The main drawback was a higher frequency of gastrointestinal side-effects[9].

The present study shows that if the new PGE analogues are used, the frequency of vomiting and diarrhoea is not higher than that with laminaria tent if the pretreatment period is 3 h. These analogues are more effective in dilating the cervical canal and the amount of blood loss is less in comparison with laminaria.

TERMINATION OF SECOND TRIMESTER PREGNANCY

Patients and methods

The study included 120 women in the 13th–24th week of pregnancy calculated from the last menstrual period and admitted to the hospital for therapeutic abortion. Before administration of the first dose of prostaglandin, a medium-size sterile laminaria was inserted into the cervical canal just beyond the internal os. The laminaria was withdrawn 12 hours later and the prostaglandin treatment commenced. The patients were then randomly divided into two treatment groups. The 64 patients in group I received 0.5 mg 16-phenoxy-ω-17,18,19,20-tetranor PGE_2 methylsulfonylamide at 4-hour intervals for up to 24 h. The 56 patients in group II were treated with 0.25 mg 15-methyl $PGF_{2\alpha}$ every second hour during the same time period. All patients received diphenoxy hydrochloride, 5 mg, three times at 4-hourly intervals starting at the same time as the first injection.

The clinical course in all patients was closely observed during the treatment by the research physician and nurses. Uterine pain was alleviated by rectal suppositories of pentazocine or intramuscular injections of meperidine (pethidine) hydrochloride. The cervix was carefully examined after the abortion for signs of rupture or laceration in all patients.

Results and comments

Both treatments were equally effective. Pretreatment with one laminaria tent for 12 h followed by intramuscular injection of 15-methyl $PGF_{2\alpha}$ or 16-phenoxy-ω-17,18,19,20-tetranor PGE_2 methylsulfonylamide resulted in an abortion within 24 hours of prostaglandin treatment in 118 out of 120 second trimester patients (98.3%). In Table 6.3 the efficacy of this treatment is compared with that of other treatments in which the vaginal or intramuscular routes are used. In all these studies the criteria for accepting the patients, the general management of the patients and definitions of success, complete abortion etc. have been the same. The results may therefore be more comparable than those of independent studies.

Table 6.3 shows that the combination of pretreatment with laminaria followed by intramuscular injections of either 15-methyl $PGF_{2\alpha}$ or 16-phenoxy-ω-17,18,19,20-tetranor PGE_2 methylsulfonylamide is more effective than if the E analogue is given alone or if E or F analogues

Table 6.3 Comparison of selected prostaglandin analogues administered by non-invasive routes for termination of second trimester pregnancy

Treatment	Frequency of abortion (%)	Mean no. of gastro-intestinal side-effects		Duration of labour (h)	Ref.
		Vomiting	Diarrhoea		
Laminaria + i.m. 15-methyl $PGF_{2\alpha}$	98.0*	0.8	0.8	10.7	3
Laminaria + i.m. 16-phenoxy PGE_2 methylsulfonylamide	98.0*	0.8	0.1	9.3	3
I.m. 16-phenoxy PGE_2 methylsulfonylamide	81.3†	1.1	0.4	15.7	10
Vaginal 9-methylene PGE_2	83.0†	0.9	0.3	15.2	11
Vaginal 15-methyl-$PGF_{2\alpha}$ me ester	80.0†	1.9	1.6	15.8	12
Vaginal 15-methyl $PGF_{2\alpha}$ me ester + i.m. 15-methyl $PGF_{2\alpha}$	93.1‡	2.8	2.1	18.6	12

* Within 24 h
† Within 30 h
‡ Within 36 h

are administered by the vaginal route. The combination of laminaria and intramuscular injections of one of the two analogues also resulted in a much shorter duration of labour, around 10 h, compared with 15–18 h for the other treatments.

Gastro-intestinal side-effects, vomiting and diarrhoea, were significantly less common if pretreatment with laminaria was combined with 16-phenoxy-ω-17,18,19,20-tetranor PGE_2 methylsulfonylamide than with 15-methyl $PGF_{2\alpha}$. Almost half of the patients (48%) did not experience any side-effects with the E analogue. The corresponding figure for the F analogue was 21% ($p < 0.005$). The mean number of episodes of vomiting and diarrhoea was 0.8 and 0.1, respectively, for the E analogue and 0.8 and 0.8, respectively, for the F analogue. Also in this respect the combination of laminaria and intramuscular injections of the E analogue compares favourably with the other alternatives. Only vaginal administration of 9-deoxo-16,16-dimethyl-9-methylene PGE_2 may compete. Therapy with this compound is, however, complicated by a higher frequency of temperature elevation.

Cervical injury has been reported to occur more frequently following prostaglandin therapy than following treatment with other compounds used for termination of second trimester pregnancy. Cervical injury is probably the result of unusual cervical resistance in the face of strong uterine contractions. The incidence of cervical tear is difficult to assess, it depends on the definition and degree of examination of the patients. When reported, the figures vary between 0.3 and 8% following prostaglandin therapy[13]. The fact that in none of the 120 patients who were treated with a combination of laminaria and intramuscular injections of a PGF or PGE analogue, a cervical laceration was observed indicates that this combination is an effective way of reducing the risk of this complication.

Conclusion

Termination of pregnancy with prostaglandin analogues offers the possibility of using non-invasive routes of administration. Non-invasive routes, e.g. vaginal or intramuscular administration, have important advantages in comparison with the intrauterine routes; inadvertant injection of the drug, e.g. into the systemic circulation, is avoided and as a result the risk of serious complications may be reduced; the simplicity of the treatment facilitates the procedure and allows extended use of paramedical personnel.

In second trimester abortions the intramuscular route may have an advantage over the vaginal one since the absorption of the drug is not influenced by an early rupture of the membranes or an early start of vaginal bleeding.

Pretreatment with laminaria followed by intramuscular injections of either 15-methyl $PGF_{2\alpha}$ or 16-phenoxy-ω-17,18,19,20-tetranor PGE_2 methylsulfonylamide seems more effective than other compounds, e.g. hypertonic saline and ethacridine lactate (Rivanol), but also more effective than natural prostaglandins and prostaglandin analogues used alone for termination of second trimester pregnancy. The PGE analogue has the advantage of a low frequency of gastro-intestinal side-effects.

Acknowledgements

The studies referred to were supported by the WHO Special Programme of Research, Development and Research Training in Human Reproduction, Geneva, Switzerland.

References

1 Bygdeman, M., Christensen, N. J., Gréen, K., Zheng, S. and Lundström, V. (1982). Termination of early pregnancy – Future development. *Acta Obstet. Gynecol. Scand.* Supp 12 (In press)

2 Christensen, N. J., Bygdeman, M. and Gréen, K. (1982). Comparison of different prostaglandin analogues and laminaria for preoperative dilatation of the cervix in late first trimester abortion. *Contraception* (In press)

3 Bygdeman, M. and Christensen, N. J. (1982). Randomized comparison between laminaria and either i.m. injection of 15-methyl $PGF_{2\alpha}$ or 16-phenoxy-ω-17,18,19,20-tetranor PGE_2 methylsulfonylamide for termination of second trimester pregnancy. *Acta Obstet. Gynecol. Scand.* (In press)

4 Fortney, J. A. and Laufe, L. E. (1978). Menstrual regulation – Risks and benefits. In Sciarra, J. J., Zatuchni, G. J. and Speidel, J. J. (eds.) *Risks, Benefits and Controversies in Fertility Control*, pp. 274–281. (Hagerstown: Harper & Row)

5 WHO Special Programme of Research, Development and Research Training in Human Reproduction. (1979). *8th Annual Report*, pp. 62. (Geneva: WHO)

6 Bygdeman, M. (1979) Menstrual regulation with prostaglandins. In Karim, S. M. M. (ed.) *Advances in Prostaglandin Research. Practical Applications of Prostaglandins and their Synthesis Inhibitors*, pp. 267–282. (Lancaster: MTP Press)

7 Karim, S. M. M. and Prasad, R. N. V. (1979). Preoperative cervical dilatation with prostaglandins. In Karim, S. M. M. (ed.) *Advances in Prostaglandin Research. Practical Applications of Prostaglandins and their Synthesis Inhibitors*, pp. 283–300. (Lancaster: MTP Press)

8 Edelman, D. A., Brenner, W. E. and Berger, G. S. (1974). The effectiveness and complications of abortion by dilatation and vacuum aspiration versus dilatation and rigid metal curettage. *Am. J. Obstet. Gynecol.*, **119**, 473

9 WHO Prostaglandin Task Force (1981). Vaginal administration of 15-methyl $PGF_{2\alpha}$ methyl ester for preoperative cervical dilatation. *Contraception*, **23**, 251

10 WHO Prostaglandin Task Force (1982). Termination of second trimester pregnancy by intramuscular injection of 16-phenoxy-ω-17,18,19,20-tetranor PGE_2 methylsulfonylamide. *Int. J. Gynecol. Obstet.*, **20**, 383

11 Bygdeman, M., Christensen, N., Gréen, K. and Lundström, V. (1980). Midtrimester abortion by vaginal administration of 9-deoxo-16,16-dimethyl-9-methylene PGE_2. *Contraception*, **22**, 153

12 WHO Prostaglandin Task force (1982). Termination of second trimester pregnancy with a long-acting vaginal pessary containing 15-methyl $PGF_{2\alpha}$ methyl ester. *Int. J. Gynecol. Obstet.* (In press)

13 Karim, S. M. M. (1979). Termination of second trimester pregnancy with prostaglandins. In Karim, S. M. M. (ed.) *Advances in Prostaglandin Research. Practical Applications of Prostaglandins and their Synthesis Inhibitors*, pp. 375–409. (Lancaster: MTP Press)

7
Clinical study of Cervagem (ONO-802) for application in first and second trimester abortions in Japan

K. SATOH, K. KINOSHITA and S. SAKAMOTO

INTRODUCTION

Prostaglandins (PGs) are routinely used for induction and augmentation of labour, since they have a strong contractile effect on the pregnant uterus. Differing from oxytocin, PGs stimulate the uterus not only in the third trimester of pregnancy but also in the first and second trimesters. Based on this, clinical application of PGs for therapeutic abortion was developed and the effectiveness of $PGF_{2\alpha}$ administered by various routes is widely recognized. However, the primary PGs produce side-effects and their duration of action is short. In order to overcome these disadvantages, the efficacy and side-effects of synthetic analogues of PGs have been studied by several investigators[1-7]. Among them, 16,16-dimethyl-*trans*-Δ^2 PGE_1 methyl ester (Cervagem, ONO-802), a PGE_1 analogue, which induces uterine contractions in rats with potency 100 times higher than that of $PGF_{2\alpha}$), was found effective for the termination of early pregnancy by intra-uterine instillation[8-9]. However, efforts have been directed towards development of simpler and more acceptable routes of administration. In 1977 Karim *et al.*[10] showed that vaginal administration of ONO-802 was effective in terminating very early pregnancy in 46 out of 50 patients with minimal side-effects. The findings have subsequently been confirmed by other investigators[11-13] in the first two trimesters of pregnancy.

The present paper describes the results of clinical studies with ONO-802 for termination of first and second trimester pregnancies in Japan.

APPLICATION IN FIRST AND SECOND TRIMESTER ABORTION

First trimester pregnancy

Patients and methods

Patients up to 12 weeks pregnant were selected in 12 university hospitals in Japan from December 1977 to July 1978. They all were desirous of undergoing therapeutic abortion under the Eugenic Protection Law and consented to be included in the study. Patients with hypersensitivity to PGs, asthma, glaucoma, severe cervicitis and colpitis were excluded.

One vaginal suppository containing 1 mg ONO-802 was administered at 3-hourly intervals up to five suppositories. The treatment, if unsuccessful, was repeated the following day.

The efficacy of the drug was judged on the following criteria. Success (complete and incomplete abortion) was confirmed by negative pregnancy test 2 weeks after drug administration. Abortion was considered complete when the products of conception could not be recovered, and incomplete when some products of conception (other than the fetus) were recovered at curettage 1 week after the treatment. When the fetus was not expelled, the treatment was considered a failure.

Cervical dilatation was measured in terms of the size of the largest Hegar dilator which could be inserted into the cervical canal without resistance.

Results

There were 110 patients in the study; 96 required a single treatment and in 14, treatment had to be repeated the following day. The patients were divided into three gestational periods: up to 6 weeks of pregnancy (15 cases), from 6 weeks to 8 weeks (40) and from 8 weeks to 12 weeks (41). Overall success rate was 91.7% (88/96) including complete (67.7%) and incomplete (24.0%) abortions. Failure rate was 8.3%

Table 7.1   Success rates of therapeutic abortion with ONO-802 suppository in the first trimester of pregnancy

Gestational age (cases)	Success % (cases)	Complete % (cases)	Incomplete % (cases)	Failure % (cases)
<6 wk (15)	93.3 (14)	80.0 (12)	13.3 (2)	6.7 (1)
6 wk 1 d–8 wk (40)	95.0 (38)	62.5 (25)	32.5 (13)	5.0 (2)
8 wk 1 d–12 wk (41)	87.8 (36)	68.3 (28)	19.5 (8)	12.2 (5)
Total (96)	91.7 (88)	67.7 (65)	24.0 (23)	8.3 (8)
Repeated administration (14)	50.0 (7)	28.6 (3)	21.4 (3)	50.0 (7)

(8/96) (Table 7.1). There were no major differences in the success rates among three groups. The success rate in the group of 14 patients in whom the treatment had to be repeated was 50% (7/14). The results indicate that a single course of administration of ONO-802 vaginal suppositories may be enough to interrupt first trimester pregnancy but there may be a few patients who are resistant to treatment with this drug.

As shown in Table 7.2, the interval between the administration of the first suppository and the onset of uterine contractions was shorter with advancing pregnancy. The same trend was found for the time of onset of bleeding after drug administration. However, the duration of bleeding (approximately 7 days) was similar in the three gestational periods.

The amount of bleeding was classified as heavy, average or scanty. Bleeding in 4.3% of the patients was heavy, 89.1% had average bleeding and 6.6% scanty. The amount of bleeding corresponded on average to the amount lost during menstruation.

The cervix had dilated up to $8.2 \, mm \pm 2.1$ (mean $\pm$ SD) from $3.3 \, mm \pm 1.5$ at 3 hours after the administration of the first pessary. The degree of dilatation in nulliparae (12 cases) and multiparae (15 cases) was from $2.3 \, mm \pm 1.3$ to $7.3 \, mm \pm 2.1$ and from $3.6 \, mm \pm 1.4$ to $8.5 \, mm \pm 1.7$, respectively (Figure 7.1). The results indicate that ONO-802 has a marked effect on the cervix and could be used as pre-treatment prior to curettage.

Side-effects observed included diarrhoea (9.7%), vomiting (7.1%), nausea (5.8%), pyrexia (> 38 °C) (3.2%), shivering (3.2%), headache (2.6%), pallor (0.7%) and lumbago (0.6%) (Figure 7.2).

Table 7.2 Therapeutic abortion in the first trimester of pregnancy with ONO-802 suppository

		Age	Gestational weeks (wk±d)	Dose (mg)	Onset of lower abdominal tension	Onset of bleeding	Duration of bleeding (d)
≦6 wk	Nulliparae (3)	26.3±11.8	5.9±0.1	5.0±0.0	6°10.7'±3°38.2'	7°55.7'±4°26.7'	6.0±4.6
	Multiparae (12)	30.2±4.5	5.5±0.4	4.6±0.8	4°14.2'±3°11.4'	6°2.9'±2°52.8'	8.0±2.4
	Total (15)	29.4±6.2	5.6±0.4	4.7±0.7	4°37.5'±3°14.7'	6°25.5'±3°9.2'	7.6±2.9
6 wk 1 d–8 wk	Nulliparae (8)	31.0±5.8	7.2±0.5	4.9±0.4	2°36.3'±1°58.3'	3°45.8'±1°26.2'	6.2±5.6
	Multiparae (32)	30.9±4.7	7.1±0.7	4.7±0.6	3°28'±1°27.7'	5°47.7'±3°17.3'	9.3±4.1
	Total (40)	30.9±4.9	7.1±0.7	4.7±0.6	3°17.4'±1°35.4'	5°27.9'±3°8.5'	8.9±4.4
8 wk 1 d–12 wk	Nulliparae (16)	25.0±8.0	10.6±1.3	4.5±1.0	3°30.5'±3°26.4'	5°11.4'±3°39.3'	5.7±5.3
	Multiparae (25)	30.7±4.7	9.7±1.2	3.5±1.6	3°26.5'±2°59.4'	4°12.5'±2°45.2'	7.9±2.9
	Total (41)	28.5±6.7	10.0±1.3	3.9±1.5	3°28'±3°7'	4°35.2'±3°7.3'	7.2±3.9

All values are mean±SD

Hegar No.

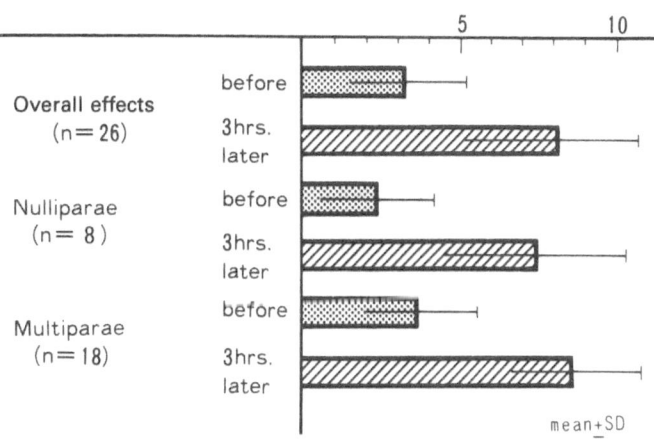

Figure 7.1 Effect of ONO-802 suppository on cervical dilatation in the first trimester of pregnancy

Frequency (%)

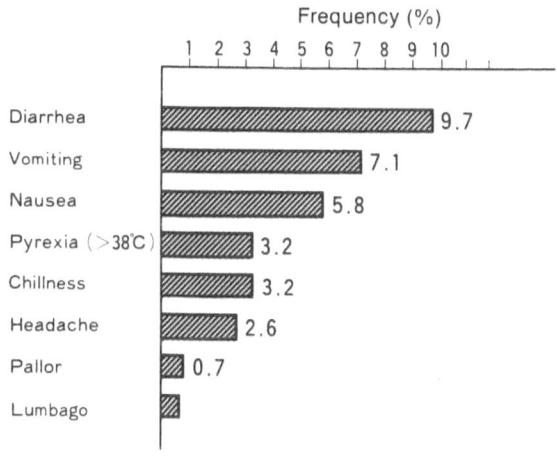

Figure 7.2 Side-effects of ONO-802 suppository in first trimester pregnancy

Second trimester pregnancy – randomized, double-blind controlled study[14, 15]

Patients and methods

The patients were selected from those (12–24 weeks) who required therapeutic abortion under the Eugenic Protection Law and consented to be included in the study. The criteria for exclusion were similar to those described before.

Two types of vaginal suppositories of the same shape and appearance were used – A: ONO-802 1.0 mg/suppository, a: placebo suppository. Appropriate packs of five A-suppositories or a-suppositories were prepared for allocation of one pack to each patient.

Random coding of the drugs was made at the control centre. The key code was kept by the controller and opened at the control centre after the completion of the study. Data analysis headquarters were set up at the Department of Obstetrics and Gynaecology, University of Tokyo, and the control centre was established by the Control Committee.

Drug administration

One of the A- or a-suppositories was inserted deep into the posterior fornix of the vagina by a forefinger without using a speculum, five times at 3-hourly intervals. Subsequent drug administration was discontinued after the onset of effective uterine contractions followed by expulsion of the products of conception.

Pelvic examination was carried out at least at 3-hourly intervals to assess progress. The efficacy was judged at 30 hours after the start of treatment, based on the following criteria: complete abortion, where both the fetus and placenta were completely expelled, and incomplete abortion, where the fetus was expelled but some products of conception (e.g. the placenta) remained in the uterus. When the drug was ineffective, the treatment was regarded as a failure. If the patient was not treated in strict accordance with the protocol, she was excluded from analysis.

If the patient failed to abort 30 h after the start of treatment, pregnancy was terminated by other methods in use at each participating institute.

Patients within the following categories were excluded from data analysis: (1) those not conforming to the criteria for selection; (2) those who underwent combined therapy with another procedure and (3) those with incomplete records.

At each insertion of the drug, the degree of cervical dilatation was measured by means of Hegar dilators changing from a large one to a smaller one.

The puerperal course, the duration of uterine bleeding and the date of onset of subsequent menstruation were recorded.

Data were analysed by the Control Committee in accordance with the Commentary to the Drug Efficacy Evaluation System. The method of analysis employed comprised U test, χ^2 test and Fisher's test.

Results

Sixty-three patients received ONO-802 suppositories and 63 the placebo. One patient in the placebo group was excluded from data analysis because she was given indomethacin suppositories during treatment with the placebo. Therefore, a total of 125 cases (63 cases in the ONO-802 group and 62 cases in the placebo group) were subjected to the data analysis.

There was no marked difference between the ONO-802 group and the placebo group in age, parity, gestational age, type of pregnancy, state of the membranes, medical complications and history of Caesarean section. It was judged that adequate randomness and balance for simple intergroup comparison by the double-blind method were maintained (Table 7.3).

Table 7.3 Characteristics of patients treated with ONO-802 suppository or placebo

	ONO-802	*Placebo*
Patient number	63	62
Age (y)	28.6 ± 5.8 (18–44)	28.7 ± 5.4 (16–43)
Parity		
Nullipara	32 (51%)	21 (34%)
Multipara	31 (49%)	41 (66%)
1	9	16
2	16	20
3	5	4
4	1	1
Gestational age (days)	128.2 ± 34.2	126.6 ± 33.5
12 wk–15 wk 6 d	24 (38%)	29 (47%)
16 wk– 19 wk 6 d	18 (29%)	12 (19%)
> 20 wk	21 (33%)	21 (34%)
Type of pregnancy		
Normal	44 (70%)	38 (61%)
Hydatidiform mole	3 (4.7%)	3 (4.8%)
Intra-uterine fetal death	10 (15.9%)	12 (19.9%)
Threatened abortion	3 (4.7%)	6 (9.5%)
Others	3 (4.7%)	3 (4.8%)
State of the membranes		
Intact	61 (97%)	60 (97%)
Ruptured	2 (3%)	2 (3%)

Source: reference 14   (mean ± SE)

The evaluation of efficacy was made in three grades: complete abortion, incomplete abortion and failed treatment. There were significantly more cases with complete and incomplete abortion in the ONO-802 group than in the placebo group (Table 7.4).

Table 7.4　Success rates of ONO-802 suppository in the second trimester of pregnancy

	Complete abortion	Incomplete abortion	Failure	Total
ONO-802	45 (71%)	10 (16%)	8 (13%)	63
	(87%)*			
Placebo	1 (2%)	0	61 (98%)	62
	(2%)*			

* $p < 0.001$
Source: reference 14

Side-effects were classified into four grades as follows: (1) none, (2) mild, not necessitating interruption of treatment, (3) side-effects that required dosing interval to be increased and (4) discontinuation of the drug due to side-effects. The incidence of side-effects was 54% in the ONO-802 group and 11% in the placebo group (Table 7.5).

Table 7.5　Side-effects with ONO-802 suppository in the second trimester of pregnancy

	No side-effects	Mild side-effects	Moderate side-effects	Discontinuation due to side-effects	Total
ONO-802	29 (46%)	29	2	3	63
		(54%)*			
Placebo	55 (89%)	7	0	0	62
		(11%)*			

* $p < 0.001$
Source: reference 14

Utility was judged on overall efficacy and safety by classifying into seven grades: very useful, fairly useful, slightly useful, not useful, slightly unfavourable, fairly unfavourable and very unfavourable. Detailed results are shown in Table 7.6.

Table 7.6 **Utility of ONO-802 suppository in the second trimester of pregnancy**

	Very useful	Fairly useful	Slightly useful	Not useful	Slightly unfavourable	Fairly unfavourable	Very unfavourable	Total
ONO-802	30 (48%)	16 (25%)	10 (16%)	5	0	1	1	63
	(89%)*					(3%)		
Placebo	0	1	0	57	2	0	2	62
	(2%)				(6%)			

* $p < 0.001$
Source: reference 14

The mean time from induction to onset of uterine contractions in 59 cases was 154.3 ± 18.1 min (mean $\pm$ SE) (7–720 min), the time to onset of bleeding in 55 cases was 323.6 ± 41.0 min (60–1,770 min), the time to fetal expulsion in 54 cases was 955.4 ± 97.0 min (150–3,090 min), and the time to placental expulsion in 54 cases was 961.6 ± 97.0 min (155–3,090 min) (Figure 7.3).

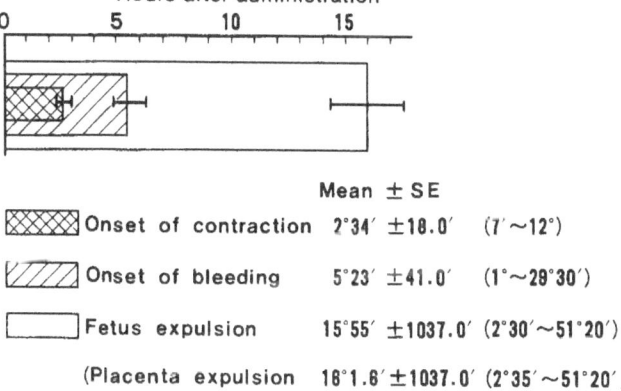

Figure 7.3 Onset time of uterine contraction and bleeding and conceptus expulsion after administration of ONO-802 suppository (second trimester pregnancy). (Source: reference 14)

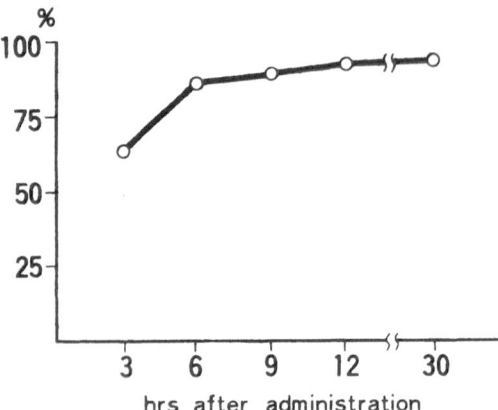

Figure 7.4 Percentages of cervical dilatation with ONO-802 suppository (second trimester pregnancy). (Source: reference 14)

The time course of cervical dilatation was studied as described before. Cervical dilatation was observed in 40 (63.5%) of 63 patients in the ONO-802 group 3 h after the start of administration. Cervical dilatation was observed in 54 cases (85.7%) at 6 h, in 56 cases (88.9%) at 9 h, and in 58 cases (92.1%) at 12 h and 30 h after the start of treatment (Figure 7.4).

The cervical canal had dilated up to 8.1 mm ± 2.1 (mean ± SD) from 3.1 ± 1.5 at 3 h after the first drug insertion in 40 cases (Figure 7.5).

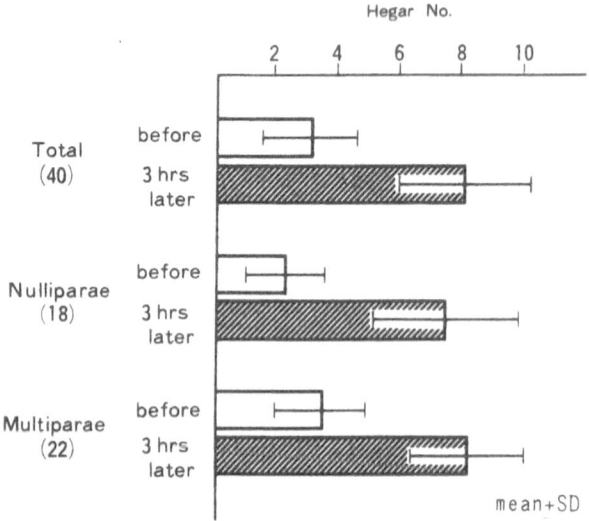

Figure 7.5 Cervical dilatation with ONO-802 suppository in second trimester pregnancy. (Source: reference 14)

The degree of the dilatation in nulliparae (18 cases) and multiparae (22 cases) was from 2.2 mm ± 1.2 to 7.5 mm ± 2.4 and from 3.4 mm ± 1.5 to 8.1 mm ± 1.9, respectively.

In the ONO-802 group, the expulsion of the fetus occurred in two (3%) of 63 cases at 3 h, in 11 cases (17.5%) at 6 h, in 15 cases (23.8%) at 9 h, in 28 cases (44.4%) at 12 h and in 55 cases (87.0%) at 30 h after the start of drug administration (Figure 7.6).

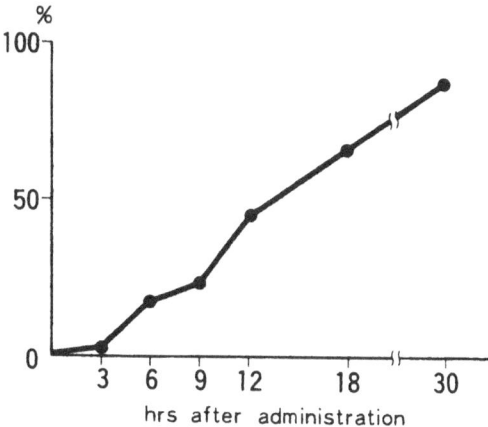

Figure 7.6 Cumulative success rates with ONO-802 suppository in second trimester pregnancy. (Source: reference 14)

The mean amount of uterine bleeding in 55 cases treated with ONO-802 was 165 ± 49 ml. The minimum blood loss was 10 ml, and blood loss of more than 500 ml was observed in three cases (5%) (600 ml, 620 ml and 2,645 ml, respectively). The case which showed the largest blood loss (2,645 ml) had a hydatidiform mole.

Side-effects included: nausea, vomiting, abdominal cramps, facial flushing, headache, dizziness, palpitation, diarrhoea and pyrexia (Table 7.7). The incidences of nausea, vomiting, abdominal cramps, diarrhoea and pyrexia were significantly higher in the ONO-802 group than in the placebo group. Discontinuation of drug administration occurred only in the ONO-802 group, i.e. in three cases which showed pyrexia (>38 °C).

Various laboratory examinations including haematological and biochemical tests on the blood revealed no significant difference between the ONO-802 group and the placebo group.

In the ONO-802 group, 62 (98%) of 63 cases showed a normal puerperal course. Only one patient developed an intra-uterine infection (due to unknown cause), but it was not a severe one. The patients in the placebo group underwent the conventional procedure for termination of pregnancy after the completion of the study. Although one patient of 62 showed uterine subinvolution, it was not severe enough to cause any problem.

In the ONO-802 group, uterine bleeding stopped within 2 weeks in 57 (90%) of 63 cases. Uterine bleeding continued for more than 2 weeks (15–38 days) in six cases, but none required any treatment. In the placebo group, after interrupting the pregnancy by the conventional method, uterine bleeding stopped within 2 weeks in 54 (87%) of 62 cases. Uterine bleeding continued for more than 2 weeks (15–21 days) in eight cases, but none required treatment.

Table 7.7 Side-effects of ONO-802 suppository in the second trimester of pregnancy

	ONO-802 (n = 63)	Placebo (n = 62)
Nausea*	17 (27.0%)	3 (4.8%)
Vomiting*	15 (23.8)	3 (4.8)
Abdominal cramps*	28 (44.4)	12 (19.4)
Flushing	14 (22.2)	6 (9.7)
Headache	12 (19.0)	5 (8.1)
Dizziness	1 (1.6)	1 (1.6)
Palpitation	3 (4.8)	2 (3.2)
Diarrhoea*	18 (28.6)	1 (1.6)
Pyrexia*	10 (15.9)	0

* $p < 0.01$
Source: reference 14

In order to estimate the endocrine state after the study, the onset of subsequent menstruation was examined by dividing into three groups, i.e. Group 1 (within 45 d), Group 2 (46–60 d) and Group 3 (after 60 d). In the case of the ONO-802 group, 51 (81%) of 63 cases fell in Group 1, seven cases (11%) in Group 2 and four cases (6%) in Group 3, one case not known. In the case of the placebo group, after terminating pregnancy by the conventional method, 46 (74%) of 62 cases fell in Group 1, ten cases (16%) in Group 2 and six cases (10%) in Group 3. The mean interval to the subsequent menstruation was 41.2 d (30–70 d) in 62 cases in the ONO-802 group and 45.3 d (24–147 d) in 62 cases in the placebo group, indicating no particular delay in onset of menstruation in either group.

Intra-uterine fetal death and hydatidiform mole

Patients and methods

Twenty-four patients with an intra-uterine fetal death (IUFD) and ten with a hydatidiform mole were treated with vaginal suppositories containing 1 mg ONO-802. The treatment schedule was the same as for first and second trimester pregnancies except that the drug insertion was stopped if abortion occurred before one course of administration was completed. The efficacy of the drug was judged on the same criteria as for the second trimester pregnancy.

Results

Success rates are shown in Table 7.8. For IUFD and molar pregnancy the success rates were 100%. The rate of complete abortion for molar pregnancy was much lower than for IUFD and normal pregnancies. As

Table 7.8   Success rates of therapeutic abortion with ONO-802 suppository

Type (cases)	Success % (cases)*	Complete % (cases)	Incomplete % (cases)	Failure % (cases)
First trimester (96)	91.7 (88)	67.7 (65)	24.0 (23)	8.3 (8)
Second trimester (63)	87.0 (55)	71.0 (45)	16.0 (10)	13.0 (8)
Intra-uterine fetal death (IUFD) (24)	100 (24)	79.2 (19)	20.8 (5)	0 (0)
Hydatidiform mole (10)	100 (10)	40.0 (4)	60.0 (6)	0 (0)
Total (193)	91.7 (177)	68.9 (133)	22.8 (44)	8.3 (16)

* Success includes complete and incomplete abortion

shown in Table 7.9, the dose of 3.2 ± 1.2 mg (mean $\pm$ SE) administered in IUFD was relatively small. The times from induction to onset of uterine contraction and bleeding in IUFD and mole were not different from that in the second trimester of pregnancy, whereas expulsion of the conceptus in IUFD and mole occurred significantly earlier than in the second trimester pregnancy ($p < 0.05$). The amount of bleeding in some cases of mole was heavy (up to 2,645 ml). Therefore, ONO-802 should be used with caution for this indication.

Table 7.9 Interruption of Intra-uterine fetal death (IUFD) and molar pregnancy with ONO-802 suppository

	IUFD	Hydatidiform mole	Second trimester pregnancies
Case no.	24	10	44
Age (y)	30.4 ± 5.5	29.7 ± 7.4	28.6 ± 5.8
Gestational weeks	20.8 ± 6.6	14.9 ± 2.5	18.3 ± 4.9
Dose (mg)	3.2 ± 1.2	4.0 ± 1.3	5.0
Onset of uterine contraction	$1° 55' \pm 49'$ $(17'-9°)$	$1° 35' \pm 18'$ $(1°-2°)$	$2° 56' \pm 23'$ $(7'-12°)$
Onset of bleeding	$4° 26' \pm 51'$ $(1°-9° 30')$	$3°38' \pm 1° 13'$ $(2°-6°)$	$8° 16' \pm 2° 41'$ $(1° 30'-29° 30')$
Expulsion of fetus	$13° 19' \pm 1° 19'*$ $(12°-14° 37')$	$9° 5' \pm 2° 8'*$	$17° 44' \pm 2°†$ $(2° 50'-51° 30')$
Expulsion of placenta	$13° 19' \pm 1° 19'*$ $(12°-14° 37')$	$(3° 15'-22° 55')$	$17° 52' \pm 2°†$ $(2° 50'-51° 30')$
Total bleeding (ml)	74.4 ± 22.5 $(20-230)$	921.7 ± 862 $(35-2,645)$	135.2 ± 21.3 $(10-620)$

$* < † \ (p < 0.05)$ (mean ± SE)

PHARMACOLOGICAL STUDIES IN CLINICAL APPLICATION

Levels of ONO-802 in plasma

The levels of ONO-802 in plasma after vaginal administration are shown in Figure 7.7. The plasma concentration of ONO-802 was measured by GC-MS in the Central Research Institute of Ono Pharmaceutical Co., Ltd. in patients who were given one suppository every 3 h containing 1 mg ONO-802. The level rapidly increased to 6.2 ± 1.5 ng/ml (mean ± SD) at 60 min after administration and thereafter decreased to 2.1 ± 0.2 ng/ml at 180 min. The second peak was detected at 60 min after the second administration. Vaginal bleeding and backache occurred 120 min after the administration of first suppository. No severe side-effects, however, occurred even when the peak values were reached.

Contraction pattern

The pattern of contraction induced by ONO-802 and recorded by the internal method are shown in Figures 7.8 and 7.9[16]. The contractions at the early stage were characterized by irregularity and low amplitude.

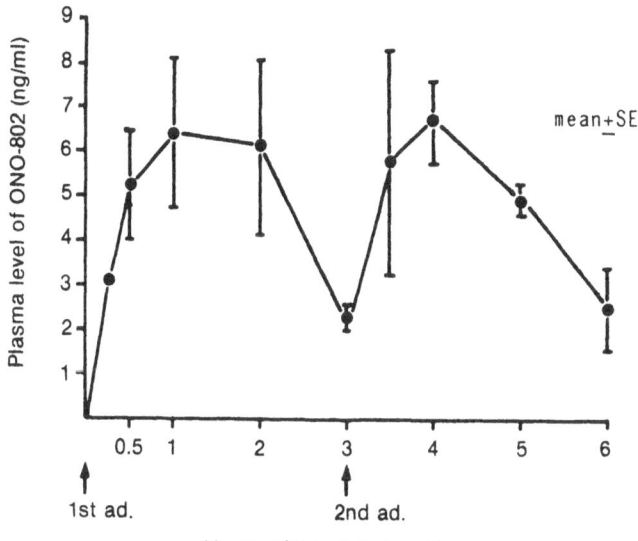

Figure 7.7 Plasma level of ONO-802 after administration of vaginal suppository

Amplitude of contractions gradually increased to 60–100 mmHg, but no elevation of intensity was observed until at the final stage.

Cervix dilating effect

Chimura and Oda[17] have studied the changes in the extensibility of human uterine cervical tissue treated with PGs. A 5.0 cm × 0.2 cm strip

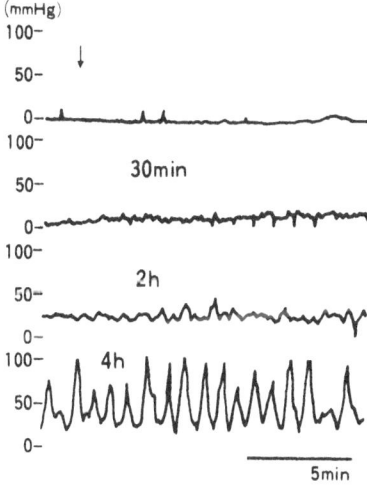

Figure 7.8 Pattern of uterine contraction with ONO-802 suppository (8 weeks of pregnancy). (Source: reference 16)

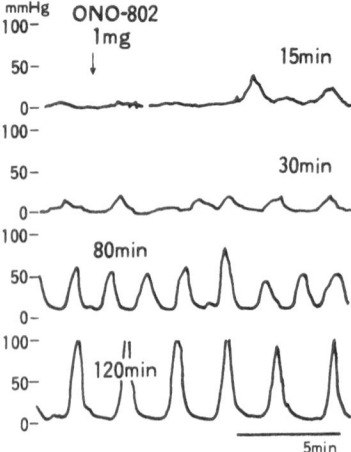

Figure 7.9 Pattern of uterine contraction with ONO-802 suppository (21 weeks of pregnancy). (Source: reference 16)

of uterine cervical tissue (2–3 months of pregnancy) was hung in Krebs–Ringer buffer and connected with a strain gauge-type transducer. Extensibility (cm/20 g/30 sec) was measured by pulling the strip with a tension of 20 g after the addition of ONO-802 (0.02 μg/ml) or PGF$_{2\alpha}$ (2.5 μg/ml) in the buffer. As shown in Figure 7.10, the extensibility with ONO-802 was almost double compared with control and was also significantly more than with PGF$_{2\alpha}$.

Mori *et al.*[18] measured the resistance pressure in dilating the cervix using a strain-gauge equipped pressure measuring device designed by them (Figure 7.11). The resistance reached 2.1 kg in dilating the cervix with Hegar No. 12 in control cases, whereas it decreased to less than half (0.9 kg) at 3 h after one ONO-802 vaginal suppository. Further-

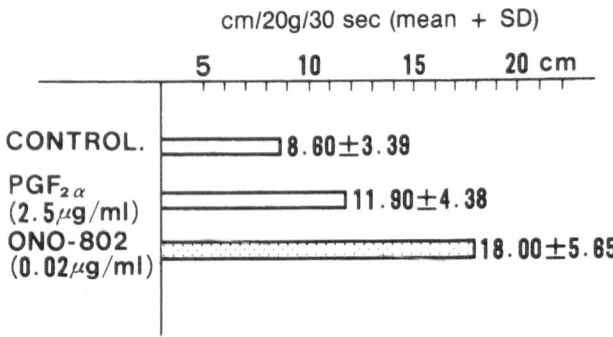

Figure 7.10 Extensibility of cervical tissue treated with ONO-802 and PGF$_{2\alpha}$. (Source: reference 17)

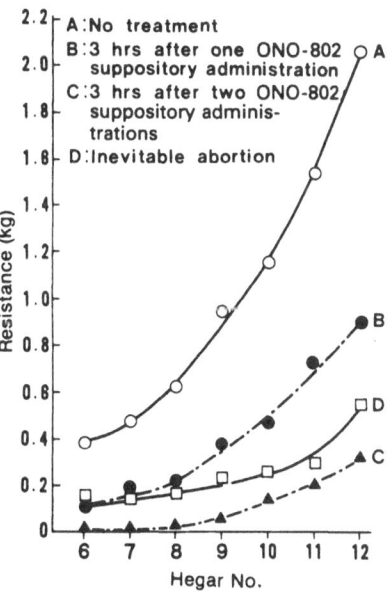

Figure 7.11   Resistance to cervical dilatation. (Source: reference 18)

more, a resistance as small as 0.3 kg (one-seventh of control) was
recorded at 3 h after the second administration. These results indicate
that ONO-802 is remarkably effective in softening or maturing the
cervix.

Levels of hormones and PGF$_{2\alpha}$ metabolite during therapeutic abortion with ONO-802 suppository

Oda *et al.*[19] measured hormone levels in plasma (estradiol-17β and progesterone) and urine (pregnanediol and hCG) in patients undergoing
first trimester abortion. As shown in Figure 7.12, plasma progesterone
started to decrease at the onset of bleeding and finally fell to 50% of the
original level at expulsion of the conceptus. Pregnanediol in urine
increased in most cases, 9–12 h after administration, but thereafter an
abrupt decrease was observed. Estradiol-17β in plasma declined
gradually and immediately after administration and reached a
significantly lower level at the onset of bleeding. These data suggest
that ONO-802 may affect steroidogenesis in the placenta. A significant
decrease in urinary hCG was observed after expulsion of the conceptus
(Figure 7.13).

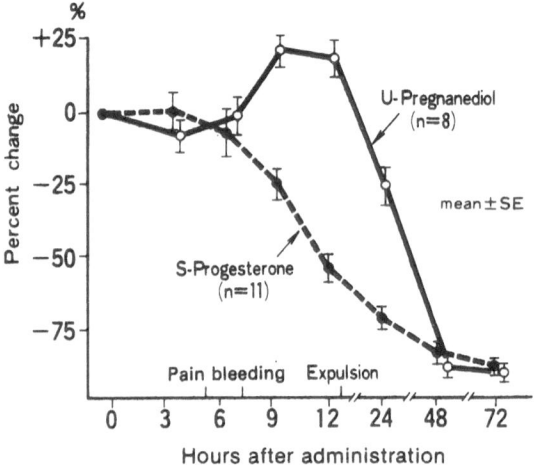

Figure 7.12 Levels of steroids during therapeutic abortion with ONO-802 suppository. (Source: reference 19)

Tominaga[20] studied the levels of the main urinary metabolite of $PGF_{2\alpha}$ ($PGF_{2\alpha}$ MUM) during abortion induced with ONO-802 suppositories. $PGF_{2\alpha}$ MUM was measured by radioimmunoassay developed by Ono Pharmaceutical Co., Ltd. As shown in Figure 7.14, changes in its urinary level were not detected during the abortion procedure. Satoh *et al.*[21] demonstrated that $PGF_{2\alpha}$ MUM level was elevated markedly during labour. On the contrary, the uterine contractions induced with ONO-802 did not result in the increased production of $PGF_{2\alpha}$.

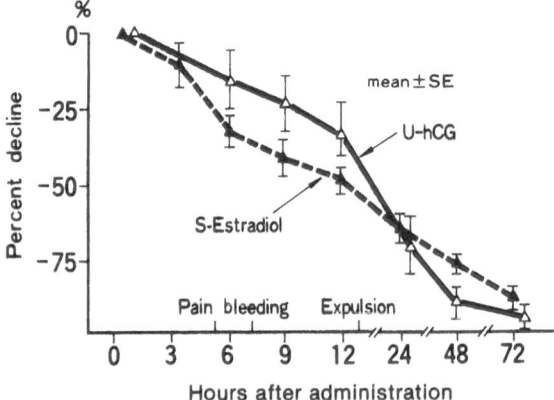

Figure 7.13 Levels of steroids and hCG during therapeutic abortion with ONO-802 suppository. (Source: reference 19)

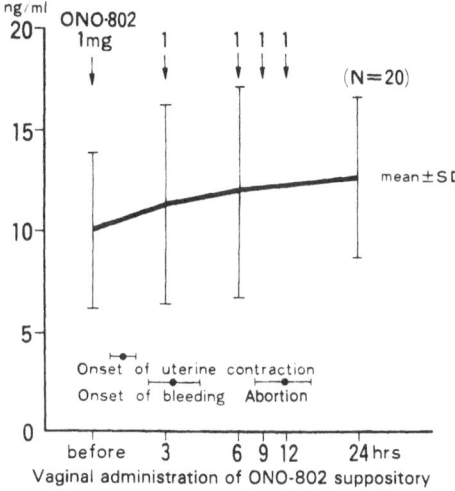

Figure 7.14 Level of $PGF_{2\alpha}$ MUM during therapeutic abortion with ONO-802 suppository. (Source: reference 20)

Physical signs during therapeutic abortion with ONO-802 suppositories

Hamada and Taki[22] recorded changes in pulse rate, blood pressure and body temperature during abortion with ONO-802 suppositories (Figure 7.15). Pulse rate and blood pressure did not change, but body temperature was elevated by 0.5 °C at 3 h after the first administration. Some patients experienced pyrexia (> 38 °C) during the procedure which occurred generally during the first 3 h.

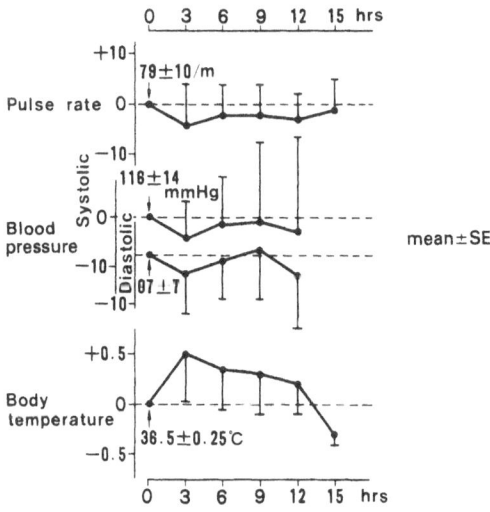

Figure 7.15 Time course of pulse rate, blood pressure and body temperature in patients given ONO-802. (Source: reference 22)

95

COMMENT

In Japan, termination of first trimester pregnancy is carried out by dilatation and curettage (D & C) or with PGs. The operative method has been in use since the termination of pregnancy was legally permitted in 1952. Sharp curettage and suction curettage are being used. PGs are also used for the termination of early pregnancy. In Japan two PGs are available for such purpose, $PGF_{2\alpha}$ (extra-amniotically) and ONO-802 (vaginally). According to Sugiyama's data[23], the average blood loss associated with sharp curettage and suction curettage at gestation up to 8 weeks was about 88 ml and 50 ml respectively. In contrast, blood loss associated with D & C (sharp curettage and suction) at 8–12 weeks' gestation increased to about 200 and 100 ml respectively. Operation time was as short as 5 min. It is evident that suction curettage has marked advantages over sharp curettage in both blood loss and operation time (Table 7.10).

Table 7.10 **Blood loss and operation time in first trimester pregnancy termination with dilatation and curettage**

	Blood loss (ml)		Operation time (min)	
Gestational weeks	Curettage	Suction	Curettage	Suction
<8 weeks	88.3 ± 17.8	49.3 ± 13.9	2.3 ± 0.2	1.4 ± 0.2
8–12 weeks	192.0 ± 79.2	110.7 ± 35.6	3.5 ± 1.0	2.3 ± 0.5

(mean ± SE)

Post-operative bleeding after D & C is usually inevitable. Duration of bleeding was reported to be 5 days in about 90% of the cases evacuated by suction curettage (Table 7.11).

Table 7.11 **Duration of post-operative bleeding in the termination of first trimester pregnancy**

	% of total cases operated	
Days after operation	Bleeding	No bleeding
up to 5 d	89.2% (669/750)	5.6% (42/750)
up to 6 d	4.4% (33/750)	0.8% (6/750)
up to 10 d	0%	

Although D & C has advantages in terms of blood loss and operation time, it is accompanied by mortality and complications such as uterine rupture, cervical laceration and anaesthetic accidents. According to the current data, the number of terminations of pregnancy was about 680,000 in 1975 in Japan. Ninety-seven percent of the cases were less than 3 months of gestation. Current data in Japan concerning the incidence of complications and mortality associated with D & C are not available. Incidence of complications was reported to be about 3.8% in 1954. Mortality rate was 0.004% during the period 1959–1965 and decreased markedly from figures reported in 1951 (Table 7.12).

Table 7.12 Incidences of complications and mortality in the termination of pregnancy

	Complications	Mortality
1951	0.3%	0.2%
	(119/39,550)	(79/39,550)
1952	2.4%	0.2%
	(154/6,405)	(13/6,405)
1953	0.8%	0.05%
	(175/21,936)	(11/21,936)
1954	3.8%	0.007%
	(4140/108,055)	(8/108,055)
1959–65		0.004%

PGs are potent abortifacient agents. In Japan we have experience with the termination of first trimester pregnancy using $PGF_{2\alpha}$, extra-amniotically and ONO-802, vaginally. $PGF_{2\alpha}$ 2–3 mg in 5 ml of saline was administered to 52 patients extra-amniotically once or twice through a Foley catheter in the hospital. In the case of ONO-802, the patients were not hospitalized, nor did they undergo D & C until 2 weeks after treatment. As a result, success rate with these two procedures was as high as about 92% (Table 7.13). There was a significant difference in the time for therapeutic abortion between ONO-802

Table 7.13 Success rates of therapeutic abortion in the first trimester of pregnancy

Treatment	Success % (cases)	Complete % (cases)	Incomplete % (cases)	Failure % (cases)
ONO-802 suppository (96)	91.7 (88)	67.7 (65)	24.0 (23)	8.3 (8)
$PGF_{2\alpha}$ (extra-amniotic) (52)	94.2 (49)	88.4 (46)	5.8 (3)	5.8 (3)

Table 7.14 Time for therapeutic abortion in the first trimester of pregnancy

Treatment	Time
ONO-802 suppository (30)	$8° 8' \pm 1° 10'$
PGF$_{2\alpha}$ (extra-amniotic) (32)	$11° 36' \pm 1° 32'$
D & C (50)	$3.1' \pm 0.6'$
ONO-802 < PGF$_{2\alpha}$ ($p < 0.01$)	(mean $\pm$ SE)

suppositories and extra-amniotic PGF$_{2\alpha}$ (Table 7.14). Blood loss was almost as much as during menstruation. It is noteworthy that the duration of bleeding of about 8 d following abortion with ONO-802 at gestation below 8 weeks was comparable to that of 6 d after D & C (Table 7.15).

Table 7.15 Comparison of ONO-802 suppository, PGF$_{2\alpha}$ (extra-amniotic) and D & C in the termination of first trimester pregnancy

	ONO-802	PGF$_{2\alpha}$	D & C
Success Rate	91.7%	94.2%	99%
Blood loss (ml)			
$\leq$ 8 wk	not less than menstruation		88.3 $\pm$ 17.8
8–12 wk			192.0 $\pm$ 79.2
Duration of bleeding (days)			
$\leq$ 8 wk	8.2 $\pm$ 3.2	8.2 $\pm$ 0.3	6
8–12 wk	7.2 $\pm$ 3.9	12.0 $\pm$ 1.4	
Side-effects	sometimes slightly	severe	
Complications (%)	not reported		3.8
Mortality (%)	not reported		0.004

(mean $\pm$ SD)

Side-effects have so far been inevitable when PGs are used for the termination of pregnancy. PGF$_{2\alpha}$ produced more severe side-effects compared with ONO-802. Premedication with analgesia was employed in patients treated with extra-amniotic PGF$_{2\alpha}$ in order to alleviate abdominal pain. ONO-802 (vaginal suppository) produced a low incidence of side-effects (except diarrhoea). Therefore, ONO-802 may be one of the recommendable abortifacients so far developed (Figure 7.16).

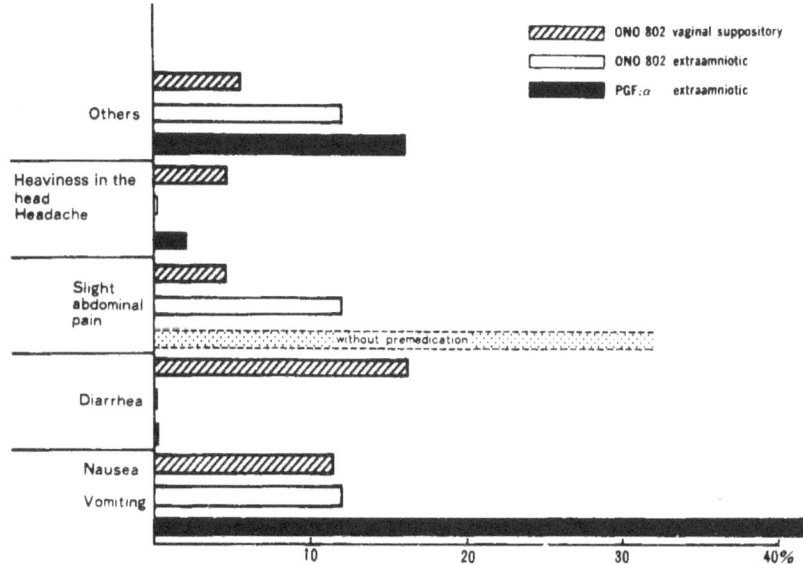

Figure 7.16   Incidences of side-effects of $PGF_{2\alpha}$ and ONO-802

D & C has advantages of very high success rate, short operation time and small amounts of blood loss, but suffers from disadvantages of 6 days' post-operative bleeding and mortality, although very low. The advantages of PGs are high success rate, small amount of blood loss and in the case of vaginal suppositories, ease of administration. The disadvantages include longer duration of bleeding and not infrequent side-effects. Thus PGs are promising abortifacients for the termination of first trimester pregnancy, although at present D & C is a common method for such a purpose in Japan (Table 7.15).

In the present study, the abortifacient effect of ONO-802 vaginal suppositories in the second trimester was investigated by the double-blind method using inactive placebo suppositories as the control drug. Some commercially available drugs were considered for selection as control drug, but only $PGF_{2\alpha}$ by extra-amniotic instillation is available in Japan. However, $PGF_{2\alpha}$ was judged unsuitable for comparison by the double-blind method, since the differences in side-effects are too large and extra-amniotic instillation would no doubt hinder the evaluation of the cervical dilating effect of ONO-802. It was therefore decided to use an inactive placebo as the control drug.

Success rates with ONO-802 suppositories and extra-amniotic $PGF_{2\alpha}$ have been similar (Table 7.16). However, the mean induction–expulsion time with ONO-802 vaginal suppositories was

Table 7.16   Success rates of therapeutic abortion in second trimester pregnancy

Treatment (cases)	Success % (cases)	Complete % (cases)	Incomplete % (cases)	Failure % (cases)
ONO-802 suppository (63)	87.0 (55)	71.0 (45)	16.0 (10)	13.0 (8)
PGF$_{2\alpha}$ (extra-amniotic) (88)	85.2 (75)	62.5 (55)	22.7 (20)	14.8 (13)

16 h, which was significantly shorter than that with PGF$_{2\alpha}$ (Table 7.17). The mean uterine bleeding was small with both methods; 165 ml with ONO-802 vaginal suppositories and 137 ml with PGF$_{2\alpha}$ (Table 7.18).

Table 7.17   Time for therapeutic abortion in the second trimester of pregnancy

Treatment	Time
ONO-802 suppository (63)	16° 2' ± 1° 37'*
PGF$_{2\alpha}$ (extra-amniotic) (88)	20° 30' ± 2° 34't
PGF$_{2\alpha}$ (i.v.) (4)	26° 23' ± 4° 30't
Oxytocin (i.v.) with laminaria (12)	25° 55' ± 3° 48't
Oxytocin (i.v.) & PGE$_2$ (per os) (2)	48° 15' ± 5° 30't
Laminaria & metreurysis (8)	70° 15' ± 8° 20't

*< t ($p < 0.001$)   (mean ± SE)

Table 7.18   Amount of bleeding associated with therapeutic abortion with ONO-802 suppository (second trimester pregnancy)

No. of cases	55
Bleeding (mean ± SE) (Range)	165 ± 49 ml (10–2645 ml)
Cases of bleeding over 500 ml	3 (600, 620, 2645 ml)

The outstanding cervical dilating effect, which had been observed in the interruption of early pregnancy[8, 11–12, 24], was confirmed as one of the characteristics of the ONO-802 vaginal suppository. It was observed that the effect reaches a plateau at about 9 h after the start of PG administration. The mechanism of action is a subject for future study, but ONO-802 may have a local effect on the uterine cervix, since in some patients cervical dilatation was without abdominal cramps due to uterine contractions. It has also been reported by Chimura et al.[17] that cervical extensibility produced by ONO-802 was more marked than with $PGF_{2\alpha}$.

With intra-uterine instillation of $PGF_{2\alpha}$, the highest incidence of side-effects were nausea and vomiting (42%), followed by pyrexia, headache and discomfort in the head, palpitation and diarrhoea. In the case of ONO-802 vaginal suppositories, abdominal cramps showed the highest incidence (44%), followed by diarrhoea, nausea, vomiting, facial flushing, headache and pyrexia. However, abdominal cramps were not severe enough to require analgesics.

The usefulness of the primary prostaglandins PGE_2 and $PGF_{2\alpha}$ for termination of pregnancy has been established. In the meantime, the development of an alternative drug with fewer side-effects and longer duration of action which can be more conveniently applied in the clinic has been undertaken. PG analogues such as 16,16-dimethyl PGE_2[2,25] and 15-methyl $PGF_{2\alpha}$ methyl ester[26,27] have been investigated using vaginal suppositories for therapeutic abortion in the second trimester. Vaginal administration of ONO-802 was demonstrated to be equally effective as 16,16-dimethyl PGE_2 and 15-methyl $PGF_{2\alpha}$ methyl ester. However, 16,16-dimethyl PGE_2 was reported to have a stability problem in suppository form[26]. Vaginal administration of 15-methyl $PGF_{2\alpha}$ methyl ester is accompanied by a moderate rate of gastro-intestinal side-effects in spite of simultaneous treatment with anti-emetics[28]. Since ONO-802 is stable in the form of a vaginal suppository which can be easily administered in the clinic and exerts outstanding clinical effects with acceptable side-effects, it may be considered superior to other analogues and may contribute to future obstetrics and gynaecology therapy.

Acknowledgements

The authors wish to express their thanks for the cooperation of 12 University Hospitals in Japan (Departments of Obstetrics and Gynaecology, University of Tokyo (Chairman: Professor S. Sakamoto), Iwate Medical College (Professor I. Nishiya), Yamagata University (Professor M. Hiroi), Niigata University (Professor S. Takeuchi), Keio University (Professor R. Iizuka), Nihon University (Professor S. Takagi), Nagoya University (Professor Y. Tomoda), Osaka University (Professor K. Kurachi), Kobe University (Professor S. Tojo), Tottori University (Professor K. Maeda), Yamaguchi University (Professor T. Torigoe) and Kyushu University (Professor

H. Nakano) for performing the clinical trials. The authors extend their thanks to Dr Koichi Yamamoto, Director of Dept of Obstetrics and Gynaecology, Tokyo Police Hospital, and Mr Tadahiro Mitsuishi, Mitsuishi Law Office, for undertaking the duties of controller, and thank the Control Committee for data analysis. The authors greatly appreciate the supply of ONO-802 vaginal suppositories for the clinical trials by Ono Pharmaceutical Co., Ltd.

References

1 Lauersen, N. H. and Wilson, K. H. (1975). Induction of mid-trimester abortion by serial intravaginal administration of 15(S),15-methyl prostaglandin $F_{2\alpha}$ (THAM) suppositories. *Prostaglandins, 10*, 1037

2 Martin, J. N., Bygdeman, M., Ramadan, M., Gréen, K., Leader, A., Lundström, V. and Wiqvist, N. (1976). Vaginally administered 16,16-dimethyl PGE_2 for the induction of mid-trimester abortion. *Prostaglandins, 11*, 123

3 Karim, S. M. M. and Ratnam, S. S. (1976). Termination of abnormal intra-uterine pregnancies with intramuscular administration of dihomo-15-methyl prostaglandin $F_{2\alpha}$. *Br. J. Obstet. Gynaecol., 83*, 885

4 Ninagawa, T., Ohta, M., Hiroshima, T., Tomita, Y., Ito, K., Imoto, N. and Matsukawa, R. (1976). Application of prostaglandin in fertility control: Japanese experience. *Proc. First Inter-Congress Asian Fed. Obstet. Gynaecol., 1*, 55

5 Sakamoto, S., Kinoshita, K. and Satoh, K. (1978). Clinical application of prosta-glandin analogs in a form of vaginal suppository for therapeutic abortion of mid-pregnancy. *Obstet. Gynecol, 44*, 691 (In Japanese)

6 Karim, S. M. M., Choo, H. T., Lim, A. L., Yeo, K. C. and Ratnam, S. S. (1978). Termination of second trimester pregnancy with intramuscular adminis-tration of 16-phenoxy-ω-17,18,19,20-tetranor PGE_2 methylsulfonylamide. *Prostaglandins, 15*, 1063

7 Kinoshita, K., Satoh, K. and Sakamoto, S. (1979). Application of 15-methyl $PGF_{2\alpha}$ methyl ester vaginal suppository for second trimester abortions. *Kanto J. Obstet. Gynaecol., 29*, 72 (In Japanese)

8 Takagi, S., Sakata, H., Yoshida, T., Nakazawa, S., Fujii, K. T., Tominaga, Y., Iwasa, Y., Ninagawa, T., Hiroshima, T., Tomida, Y., Itoh, K. and Matsukawa, R. (1977). Termination of early pregnancy by ONO-802 (16,16-dimethyl-*trans*-Δ^2 PGE_1 methyl ester). *Prostaglandins, 14*, 791

9 Karim, S. M. M. and Ratnam, S. S. (1977). Newer aspects of practical appli-cations of prostaglandins in obstetrics and gynaecology. In Karasch, N. and Fried, J. (eds.) *Biochemical Aspects of Prostaglandins and Thromboxanes. Proceedings of Intra-Science Research Foundation Symposium, Dec. 1–3, 1976*, p. 115. (New York: Academic Press)

10 Karim, S. M. M., Ratnam, S. S. and Illancheran, A. (1977). Menstrual induction with vaginal administration of 16,16-dimethyl-*trans*-Δ^2 PGE_1 methyl ester (ONO-802). *Prostaglandins, 14*, 615

11 Takagi, S., Sakata, H., Yoshida, T., Den, K., Fujii, K., Amemimya, H. and Tomita, M. (1978). Termination of early pregnancy by ONO-802 suppositories (16,16-dimethyl-*trans*-Δ^2 PGE_1 methyl ester). *Prostaglandins, 15*, 913

12 Wagatsuma, T., Tabuchi, T., Tabei, T. and Kaku, R. (1979). Interruption of pregnancy with vaginal suppositories containing 16,16-dimethyl-*trans*-Δ^2 prosta-glandin E_1. *Contraception, 19*, 591

13 Satoh, K., Kinoshita, K., Yasumizu, T. and Sakamoto, S. (1978). Application of ONO-802 vaginal suppository for first and second trimester abortions. *Kanto J. Obstet. Gynaecol.*, **27**, 132 (In Japanese)

14 Sakamoto, S., Satoh, K., Kinoshita, K., Nishiya, I., Kunimoto, K., Hiroi, M., Chimura, T., Oda, T., Hasegawa, T., Takeuchi, S., Satoh, Y., Iizaka, R., Kobayashi, T., Takagi, S., Yoshida, T., Sakata, T., Tomoda, Y., Ninagawa, T., Kurachi, K., Tanizawa, O., Hisa, Y., Tojo, S., Mochizuki, M., Maeda, K., Tominaga, Y., Mio, Y., Torigoe, T., Koresawa, M., Migita, M., Taki, I. and Hamada, T. (1981). Application of ONO-802 for second trimester abortion – double blind controlled study. *Obstet. Gynecol.*, **48**, 1681 (In Japanese)

15 Sakamoto, S., Satoh, K., Nishiya, I., Kunimoto, K. *et al.* Abortifacient effect and uterine cervix-dilating action of 16,16-dimethyl-*trans*-Δ^2 PGE$_1$ methyl ester (ONO-802) in the form of a vaginal suppository (a randomized, double-blind, controlled study in the second trimester of pregnancy). *Prostaglandins Leukotrienes Med.*, **9**, 349

16 Ohkawa, R. (1982). A study on the uterine contractile effect of 16,16-dimethyl-*trans*-Δ^2 PGE$_1$ methyl ester (ONO-802). *Acta Obstet. Gynaecol. Japn.*, **34**, 460 (In Japanese)

17 Chimura, T. and Oda, T. (1980). Effect of ONO-802 on the cervical canal and uterine blood flow. *Obstet. Gynaecol. Ther.*, **41**, 721 (In Japanese)

18 Mori, T., Watanabe, S. and Takahashi, S. (1980). A newly designed device for measurement of the resistance pressure in dilating the cervix and its application in early pregnancy. *World Obstet. Gynaecol.*, **32**, 505 (In Japanese)

19 Oda, T., Chimura, T. and Hiroi, M. (1979). Studies on the abortifacient effect of ONO-802 on early pregnancy and hormone levels in the administration. *Obstet. Gynecol.*, **46**, 1651 (In Japanese)

20 Tominaga, Y. (1979). Therapeutic abortion with PGE$_1$ analog vaginal suppository. *Obstet. Gynaecol. Ther.*, **39**, 983 (In Japanese)

21 Satoh, K., Yasumizu, T., Fukuoka, H., Kinoshita, K., Kaneko, Y., Tsuchiya, M. and Sakamoto, S. (1979). Prostaglandin F$_{2\alpha}$ metabolite levels in plasma, amniotic fluid, and urine during pregnancy and labor. *Am. J. Obstet. Gynecol.*, **133**, 886

22 Hamada, T. and Taki, I. (1980). The abortifacient effect of prostaglandin E$_1$ analogue by vaginal administration in midtrimester pregnancy. *World Obstet. Gynaecol.*, **32**, 713 (In Japanese)

23 Sugiyama, S. (1980). Personal communication

24 Nakano, R., Hata, H., Sasaki, K. and Yamoto, M. (1980). The use of prostaglandin E$_1$ analogue pessaries in patients having first trimester induced abortions. *Br. J. Obstet. Gynaecol.*, **87**, 287

25 Karim, S. M. M. (1977). Termination of pregnancy with vaginal administration of 16,16-dimethyl prostaglandin E$_2$ p-benzaldehyde semicarbazone ester. *Br. J. Obstet. Gynaecol.*, **84**, 135

26 Gréen, K. and Bygdeman, M. (1976). Plasma levels of the methyl ester of 15-methyl PGF$_{2\alpha}$ in connection with intravenous and vaginal administration. *Prostaglandins*, **11**, 879

27 Bygdeman, M., Gauguli, A., Kinoshita, K. and Lundström, V. (1977). Development of a vaginal suppository suitable for single administration for interruption of second trimester pregnancy. *Contraception*, **15**, 129

28 Bygdeman, M., Borell, U., Leader, A., Lundström, V., Martin, J. N. Jr., Eneroth, P. and Gréen, K. (1976). Induction of first and second trimester abortion by the vaginal administration of 15-methyl PGF$_{2\alpha}$ methyl ester. In Samuelson, B. and Paoletti, R. (eds.) *Advances in Prostaglandin and Thromboxane Research*. Vol. 2, pp. 693–704. (New York: Raven Press)

Discussion 3

(14) **Dr Satoh** (Japan): You used laminaria tents for decreasing duration of abortion besides decreasing the incidence of cervical laceration. How many laminaria did you use?

Dr Bygdeman: We used only one medium-sized laminaria tent 12 hours prior to PG administration. We had at least 120 patients in our study and have not encountered problems in introducing or removing the laminaria.

(15) **Dr Satoh:** Did you measure cervical dilatation after laminaria insertion?

Dr Bygdeman: No, not for second trimester abortion. The only information we have is that the diameter of the laminaria tent when you take it out is around 10 mm. The degree of dilatation will be at least that and possibly a little more than 10 mm.

Dr Fylling: Have you recorded any increase in the incidence of infection with laminaria tent?

Dr Bygdeman: The background to our use of laminaria was the discussion in the WHO PG Task Force and we were of course concerned about the risk of infection. Some pilot studies were therefore performed here in Singapore by Dr Karim and also by Dr Charles Ballard in Los Angeles. The results of these pilot studies, as well as of other studies, published in the literature, indicate that with modern laminaria which are sterilized effectively, there is no increase in infection rate if the pre-treatment time is restricted to 12 hours and the preferable time, we found, is between 8 and 12 hours.

We screen all our abortion patients for gonorrhoea and other infections and if we have a positive culture the patients will be treated with antibiotics before abortion.

(16) **Dr Puraviappan** (Malaysia): May I know how you went about terminating second trimester pregnancies – in those cases where you have failed with PGs?

Dr Bygdeman: Well, there were two cases which were regarded as failures. One was with 15-methyl $PGF_{2\alpha}$. She got a lot of gastro-intestinal side-effects following the first injection and we switched over to Sulprostone and she aborted uneventfully 12 hours later. In the second case, there was an allergic reaction to PG treatment. That resolved in 12 hours. At the same time, we had given the patient pethidine and also chlorpromazine. We re-started treatment with PG after 12 hours with a small dose and increased the dose and found that she was not allergic to PG but probably to some of the other drugs she was given. She aborted uneventfully.

Dr Karim: I will make a comment on failed treatment. This happens sometimes and there is a temptation to resort to surgery if the patient fails to abort within a specified time. If I talk in general terms about up to 10,000 second trimester abortions that have been performed in Singapore in the past 10 years with PGs, the number of patients who have ended up with surgery for failed PG treatment would be less than ten. In some of them, surgery could have been avoided as there are several alternatives available in case treatment fails. The problem that arises often is that if you have given PGs intra-amniotically and the patient fails to abort, say, within 24 hours and during that time membranes have ruptured, a repeat intra-amniotic dose is not possible. In that case, one can resort to extra-amniotic or intramuscular treatment. Some of you may be faced with the problem that you do not have an alternative available in the form of another PG or even the same

105

PG cannot be administered by other routes. In this case, one can often resort to conventional treatment, that is, use of oxytocin. If the abortion process has proceeded sufficiently – if there is progress – there is cervical dilatation, but the patient has failed to abort, quite often the use of high concentration oxytocin given intravenously will complete the process and it is very rarely necessary to resort to surgery.

Dr Bygdeman: I completely agree. As I can remember I have only had one case of surgery and that was for a uterine rupture. Otherwise, when we don't have analogues we use oxytocin.

(17) **Dr Choong Kuo Hsiang:** I am sorry to interrupt this agreement between the two experts. It would appear to me, Professor Bygdeman, that the use of laminaria tent with its advantages of decreased bleeding and so on is a backward step. After all our philosophy is to try to make the method as simple as possible. I think going back to laminaria tent with its risks of infection and so on is just making things a bit more complex. You have any comments on that?

Dr Bygdeman: I agree with that. The reason why we included laminaria tent in the pre-operative cervical dilatation study is that it is the major method used in the United States to achieve cervical dilatation prior to D & C. We wanted to see how it compared with PGs. I agree that for pre-operative cervical dilatation, PGs offer advantage over laminaria tent. When we come to second trimester abortion, the situation is somewhat different where the combination of laminaria and PGs seems to be very effective and is, as far as I can see now, the only way to reduce the frequency of cervical laceration and also obtain a short duration of labour.

(18) **Dr Sivasamboo:** I was just wondering – supposing we took this laminaria tent and before insertion soak it in sterilized saline and insert it, would we be able to reduce the number of hours required?

Dr Bygdeman: I don't know. In the United States, they have developed an alternative to laminaria to achieve cervical dilatation more rapidly than with the ordinary laminaria tent. I have not seen any results yet.

Dr Karim: The cervical dilators are made from magnesium sulphate and it is claimed that they absorb moisture much faster than natural laminaria tents.

(19) **Dr Khew:** I see that Ono has come out with a suppository for the vagina, but repeated vaginal examinations of the patient, inserting it every 3 hours, may not be too practical, as far as infection is concerned. Have you ever thought of using suppositories by the rectal route and what is the contraindication for that?

Dr Satoh: Of course, repeated vaginal examination will increase infection but this is a clinical trial. That is why we had to carry out vaginal examination frequently. In clinical use we don't have to do that – repeated vaginal examination.

We could use the suppository *per rectum* but according to some basic data, PGs are more effectively absorbed from the vagina. That is why I think vaginal administration is much better than rectal. Besides, sometimes diarrhoea happens after administration of ONO-802. If we put the suppository in the rectum, and the patient has diarrhoea, the suppository may be expelled.

(20) **Dr Guna** (Kuala Lumpur, Malaysia): Is it really necessary that the vaginal pessary should be inserted deep into the posterior fornix or could it just be pushed into the vagina? The reason why I am asking is that if it is not necessary to be inserted into the posterior fornix, then a nurse with minimal training can administer it.

Dr Satoh: In our trials, we don't use any speculum, any instrument to open the vagina, we just use the fingers. The suppository is pushed into the vagina as deep as possible. Although we didn't make sure where the suppository was, the effects were satisfactory.

(21) **Dr Simandjuntak:** In Indonesia, we also use ONO-802 for termination of abnormal pregnancy including mole. In your series, I have seen one case of bleeding with more than 2000 ml blood loss and also an average nearly 1 litre, but the efficacy is very good – 100%. We find it also the same but the bleeding is not as high as you have reported. This mole is a problem in our university. The frequency is high. We want to know what your comment is. Is there a contraindication for the use of Cervagem for evacuating a mole?

Dr Satoh: Prostaglandins can be used to expel the mole but we should exercise caution because we have seen a large amount of bleeding during abortion of hydatidiform mole. Besides, the onset of bleeding is very early, much earlier than in the normal pregnancy, and is continuous.

Dr Bygdeman: I disagree a little with you in this respect. It is my opinion that PGs administered by non-invasive routes, like the vaginal or intramuscular, are very valuable when you treat patients with hydatidiform mole and missed abortion or intra-uterine death. When compared with other methods, PGs for this type of treatment are very valuable and superior. In our department, at least, PGs are the first choice in patients with an advanced molar pregnancy and in cases of fetal death. If it is a molar pregnancy before the 12th week, I agree with you that you can use the vacuum aspiration procedure, but after the 12th week, we prefer prostaglandin treatment followed by vacuum aspiration.

Dr Satoh: But I disagree a little with you in the case of hydatidiform mole because in our department, even after abortion by PGs, we use curettage to complete the expulsion of hydatidiform mole. If we compare the time of abortion between PGs and D & C, the time for D & C is much shorter than PGs. We are using PGs for hydatidiform mole but sometimes I think D & C is better than PGs in the case of hydatidiform mole.

(22) **Dr Teo:** How do you differentiate between complete and incomplete abortion? I think it is quite easy, particularly in the second trimester, to decide, but what are your criteria for deciding whether it is complete or not, in the first trimester?

Dr Crowshaw: In most of the trials, we rely heavily on hCG determination. The investigators use an estimate of a low or zero titre of hCG after a certain period after the procedure (either 1 or 2 weeks) and their previous experience allows them to then judge whether the abortion is complete or not on that basis.

Dr Satoh: In Japan, we differentiate between complete and incomplete abortion by a different method. One week after treatment, we confirm uterine content by curettage. If there is some amount of placenta still remaining in the uterus 1 week after D & C or aspiration, we call it incomplete abortion, but the success rate is usually designated by negative pregnancy test 2 weeks after treatment.

Dr Crowshaw: I will make an additional point about that. Most of the May & Baker clinical trials have been in very early pregnancy (up to 2 weeks' overdue menstruation) and it is difficult to see very, very small amounts of residual products of conception, so it was not felt justified to do our trials that way. That is why we rely heavily on hCG determination.

8
Cervagem clinical trials review. Part 2: second trimester therapeutic termination of pregnancy, and other applications

K. CROWSHAW

INDUCTION OF SECOND TRIMESTER ABORTION

In addition to the comprehensive studies by Dr Satoh and his colleagues (presented in Chapter 7), five other centres in Japan have participated in a clinical trial programme to evaluate the use of ONO-802 in the termination of second trimester pregnancy. All six studies have been published[1-6]. Dr Satoh was analyst in the first study which was a multicentre double-blind controlled study organized by Professor Sakamoto. The other five studies are uncontrolled.

We at May & Baker have analysed the results obtained from all six centres in a uniform manner consistent with the methods used in our own trials. This analysis is shown in Table 8.1. Of 203 patients who were treated with ONO-802, 22 patients were withdrawn from the analysis for various reasons. For example, one patient (Centre 2) was misdosed at the start of the trial. Seven patients (Centre 4) had co-therapy with metreurynter, $PGF_{2\alpha}$ and/or oxytocin, and another patient (Centre 4) was diagnosed placenta praevia. In Centre 5, 11 patients were withdrawn due to co-treatment with laminaria, and two because their gestational age was greater than 28 weeks. Overall, 135 (74.6%) patients had a complete abortion. Another 25 (13.8%) had incomplete abortions, and placental tissue had to be removed by

Table 8.1 ONO-802: second trimester termination of pregnancy. Analysis of results from six Japanese centres

Trial centre	Stage of pregnancy (weeks)	Number of patients				Efficacy		
		Entered	Receiving ONO-802	Withdrawn	Analysed	Complete	Incomplete	Failure
1	>12	126	63	0	63	45/63	10/63	8/63
2	12–23	44	20	1	19*	15/19	4/19	0
3	12–26	30	30	0	30†	21/30	2/30	7/30
4	13–29	23	23	8	15	12/15	3/15	0
5	13–26	42	42	13	29‡	24/29	2/29	3/29
6	12–23	25	25	0	25	18/25	4/25	3/25
	Total	290	203	22	181	135/181	25/181	21/181
					(%)	74.6	13.8	11.6

* 4 were IUFD with no failure (all complete)
† 4 were IUFD with one failure of treatment
‡ 9 were IUFD with no failures (one incomplete)

curettage. Twenty-one (11.6%) were failures and other methods were employed to effect abortion.

It is interesting to examine some sub-groups of patients in these trials (see footnote on Table 8.1). In Chapter 7 Dr Satoh presented some data on the use of ONO-802 in some cases where intra-uterine fetal deaths (IUFD) were diagnosed. In Centre 2, four cases were IUFD and from that group there were no failures of treatment. In Centre 3, another four were IUFD and there was one failure. Lastly, there were nine IUFD in Centre 5. There were no failures but one was classified as incomplete abortion.

The most commonly reported side-effects, as other speakers have mentioned, were diarrhoea, vomiting and nausea (Table 8.2). These are the side-effects most commonly associated with prostaglandin therapy. However, the majority of cases were single incidences and the episodes were generally mild. Pyrexia was seen in 19 patients (11%). Some other side-effects were less frequently seen. In two patients treatment was discontinued due to a fall of blood pressure after the start of drug treatment[3].

A comparative study between saline instillation and ONO-802 vaginal pessaries for second trimester abortion has been carried out by Dr Affandi and his co-workers in Indonesia[7]. We are fortunate to have a number of his colleagues here today. The results of this trial cannot be compared directly with the previously discussed trials due to

Table 8.2 ONO-802: second trimester termination of pregnancy. Analysis of side-effects from six Japanese centres (181 patients)

Side-effects	Number of reports	%
Diarrhoea	36	20
Vomiting	29	16
Lower abdominal pain	28	16
Nausea	25	14
Pyrexia	19	11
Flushing	16	9
Headache	16	9
Palpitations	3	2
Dizziness	2	1
Fall of blood pressure*	2	1
Transient tachycardia	1	0.5

* This was the only side-effect leading to discontinuation of drug administration (2 patients)

differences in study design. In this study, in the event of abortion not having occurred with 24 h after ONO-802 or saline treatment, intravenous oxytocin was administered. In addition, if abortion had not taken place in either group within 48 h after the start of oxytocin infusion, the treatment was considered to be unsuccessful and other methods of abortion were undertaken.

The average time for abortion in the ONO-802 group was just over half that for the saline group (Table 8.3). There were two failures in each group. The incidence of side-effects was generally low. Diarrhoea and/or vomiting were seen in four of the 50 ONO-802 treated patients compared to none in the saline treated group. Interestingly, fever was noted in both groups – two being reported in the saline group and three in the ONO-802 treated group.

Table 8.3 Time course of abortion induced by ONO-802 or hypertonic saline in second trimester pregnancies

	Minimum		Abortion time Maximum		Average		Failures
	h	min	h	min	h	min	
ONO-802	4	10	34	21	17	49	2/50
Saline	6	12	52	39	32	17	2/50

Source: reference 7

USE OF CERVAGEM IN OTHER INDICATIONS

I would now like to discuss some of the confirmed uses and some of the potential uses for ONO-802. We have heard presentations on the use of Cervagem for the termination of second trimester pregnancy and for pre-operative cervical dilatation in pregnant women. In addition, we are currently looking at its use in non-pregnant women for dilatation of the cervix prior to operations such as diagnostic curettage and cervical biopsy. Some clinicians have also expressed interest in using Cervagem for the investigation and treatment of infertility in women. Although these studies in non-pregnant women have started, full results were not available in time for this symposium. However, preliminary comments from one of the participating clinicians do indicate that Cervagem can induce cervical dilatation in non-pregnant women although there have been a few patients who have failed to respond.

First trimester abortion

A considerable number of clinical trials have been carried out in Japan and in numerous other countries worldwide on the use of Cervagem for the induction of first trimester abortion, and some of these studies have already been mentioned by previous speakers. I will briefly review the results of just two of these trials.

One of the earliest published studies was by Takagi et al.[8] in 1978. Forty-five patients were treated with pessaries containing 0.5 mg of ONO-802 and eight patients were given pessaries with 1 mg of ONO-802 (Table 8.4). Their stage of pregnancy was from 11 to 66 days beyond the last expected menstrual period, with an average of 24 days. The success rate using the larger dose was high (89%) and side-effects were no more serious at this dose. An interesting facet of these studies was that, in five patients, serial samples of antecubital blood were taken to monitor changes in three plasma steroids, oestradiol,

Table 8.4   Termination of early pregnancy with ONO-802 suppositories

Dose	Treated	Complete	Incomplete	Failures
			Number of patients*	
0.5 mg 3-hourly	45	28 (84%)	7 (16%)	0
1.0 mg 3-hourly	18	16 (89%)	2 (11%)	0

* Administration discontinued after the onset of vaginal bleeding. Not all patients received the full course of five suppositories
Source: reference 8

progesterone and 17α-hydroxyprogesterone, during treatment. Although the fall in steroid levels was erratic during the first 24 h, all steroid concentrations fell to low levels at 48 h, consistent with termination of pregnancy.

Another of the early dose-ranging studies was carried out by Professor Karim here in Singapore[9]. Two dose regimens were studied. High success rates were obtained when early pregnant patients were treated every 4 hours with pessaries containing 1 mg ONO-802. Every patient received a total of five pessaries. In these patients, levels of plasma steroids and hCG (human chorionic gonadotrophin) were monitored at 2, 4, 8, 12 and 24 hours following administration of the first pessary (Figure 8.1). In these six patients, in whom abortion was induced, hCG, 17α-hydroxyprogesterone, oestradiol and progesterone levels all decreased steadily with 24 h. The success rate for patients treated with 0.5 mg ONO-802 pessaries 3-hourly was less good. Figure 8.2 shows the results of plasma assays from four patients who failed to respond to the lower dose regimen. There was no decrease in hCG or steroid levels within 24 h. These results were consistent with a failure to induce abortion.

From these and similar studies, it was concluded that the most acceptable dose regimen for early abortion, with both a high success rate and a moderate level of side-effects, was the 3-hourly administration of 1 mg ONO-802 pessaries. The maximum sequential administration should be five pessaries over a 12-hour period. There have been a large number of clinical studies using this dose regimen and I shall summarize results obtained from two of them.

The first is the multicentre study carried out by the World Health Organization[10]. Professor Bygdeman in Stockholm was the clinical coordinator of this study and other participating centres were based in India, Switzerland, Cuba, Hong Kong, Russia, Yugoslavia, Norway and Singapore. Three of the investigators involved in this study are attending this conference. Besides Professor Bygdeman, we have Professor Karim and Dr Fylling. Although Professor Ma could not attend due to a prior engagement in the United States, her colleague, Dr Ho, is here and has presented data on cervical dilatation (Chapter 4).

Table 8.5 summarizes the results of this WHO study. The study included 358 early pregnant women with a mean gestational age of 7 weeks. The maximum duration of amenorrhoea was 56 days. All patients received a full course of five pessaries, one administered every 3 hours, over a 12-hour period. Although a cause for concern was the 5.6% failure rate and the 8.4% of incomplete abortions requiring

114

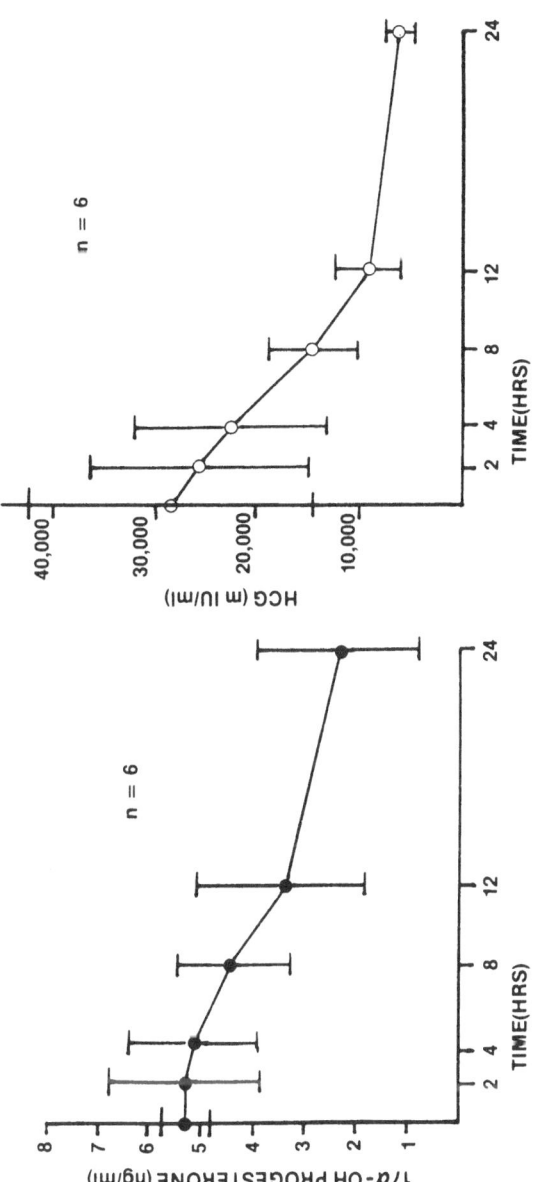

Figure 8.1 Plasma levels of 17α-OH progesterone and hCG in patients following administration of 1 mg ONO-802 pessaries. Six patients were treated 4-hourly, a total of five pessaries being administered. All were successfully aborted

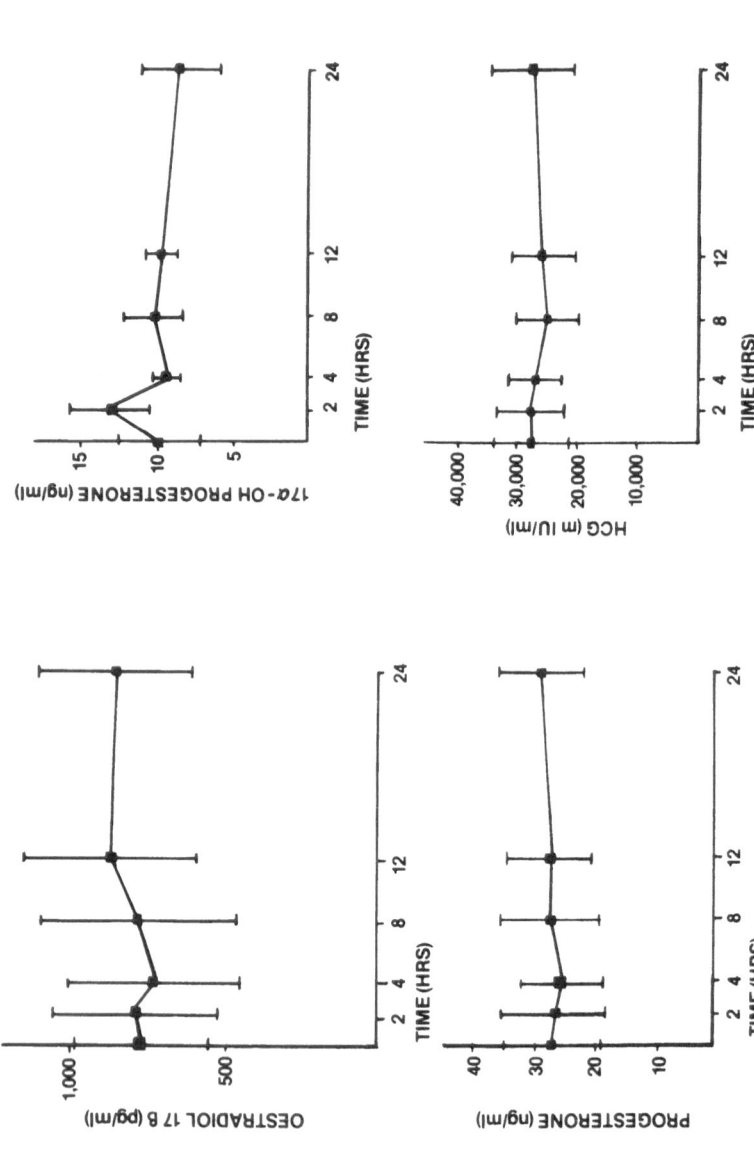

Figure 8.2 Plasma steroid and urinary hCG levels in four patients following administration of 0.5 mg ONO-802 pessaries (five over 12 hours). All four patients failed to abort

Table 8.5 ONO-802: termination of early pregnancy. WHO multicentre study

Patients treated with ONO-802	Complete	Incomplete	Failure
358	308 (86%)	30 (8.4%)	20 (5.6%)

Side-effects	Incidence
Pain	104 (29%)
Diarrhoea	96 (27%)
Vomiting	85 (24%)
Pelvic infection	9 (2.5%)
Mild pyrexia	1 (0.3%)

follow-up curettage, this does not diminish the otherwise excellent results obtained, including the 86% success rate in inducing complete abortion. Compared to other prostaglandin analogues, ONO-802 caused a relatively low incidence of the expected side-effects, namely pain, vomiting and diarrhoea. One other interesting facet of this study was the relatively low incidence of pyrexia, with just one case reported.

Similar results to these were obtained by Dr Smith and Professor Baird who carried out a similar trial on a smaller scale in Edinburgh[11]. In this study, 30 patients were treated with ONO-802, and the results were compared with those of suction termination under both local and general anaesthesia (Table 8.6). Four failures of treatment occurred in both the ONO-802 group and in the suction termination group under local anaesthetic. It is important to note the value of conducting hCG determinations as a test for continued pregnancy at 2 weeks *and* 4 weeks after treatment. For example, in the ONO-802 group, ten were positive at 2 weeks, but at 4 weeks only four were still positive by this test. An attempt to assess pain associated with the three treatments was

Table 8.6 Termination of early pregnancy. A comparison of ONO-802 and suction termination

Treatment	Anaesthetic	Pregnancy test after termination 2 weeks +ve	2 weeks −ve	4 weeks +ve	4 weeks −ve
ONO-802 (n = 30)	None	10	20	4*	26
Suction (n = 28)	Local	7	21	4*	24
Suction (n = 28)	General	1	27	0	28

* All patients had a diagnostic curettage
Source: reference 11

also made in this study (Table 8.7). There was no clear-cut difference between the three procedures, although more severe pain did appear to be associated with suction termination under local anaesthetic compared to general anaethesia, with ONO-802 lying somewhere between.

Although we are encouraged by the results of these trials, we feel that in the development of any treatment for the termination of early pregnancy we should strive to minimize the incidence of failed or incomplete abortions. We are currently examining the possibility of using controlled-release vaginal pessaries which will optimize the release of ONO-802, that is to say at a rate high enough to produce abortion but below that which would produce unacceptable levels of pain or side-effects associated with prostaglandin administration. Although work is progressing well we are not able on this occasion to present clinical trial results to you.

Table 8.7   Abdominal pain after three different termination procedures

Treatment	Severity of pain, compared with menstrual pains		
	Less severe	Similar	More severe
ONO-802	14	6	10
Suction, local anaesthesia	12	2	14
Suction, general anaesthesia	10	7	11

Source: reference 11

Menstrual regulation

I should now like to make a few comments about menstrual regulation. In women who have regular periods, an overdue period in the majority of cases is due to pregnancy. Any technique used at that time to terminate pregnancy and induce menstrual bleeding would be described as menstrual regulation. Menstrual regulation can be achieved by the vaginal administration of Cervagem. One of the earliest studies in this indication was conducted by Professor Karim[12], here in Singapore. The number of patients studied was 50 (Table 8.8). The criterion for patient selection was delayed menstruation for up to 2 weeks. Vaginal pessaries containing 1 mg of ONO-802 were administered at 4-hourly intervals to a maximum of five doses. The criteria for successful treatment were onset of uterine bleeding after prostaglandin administration and a negative pregnancy test within 2 weeks of prostaglandin administration.

Table 8.8. **Menstrual regulation with vaginal administration of ONO-802**

Number of patients:	50
Criterion for patient selection:	Delay in menstruation of up to 2 weeks
Drug:	ONO-802 vaginal pessaries
Dose:	1.0 mg 4-hourly (maximum 5 doses)

Criteria for successful treatment
Onset of uterine bleeding after prostaglandin administration and a negative pregnancy test within 2 weeks of PG administration

Source: reference 12

On admission, the women underwent an hCG test for pregnancy and, although the results were not available until 24 hours later, it did enable the following analysis of the results (Table 8.9). Of the 50 cases, treatment was successful overall in 46 patients (92%). Of the 19 patients with negative pregnancy tests initially, all responded with menstrual bleeding. This is a rather interesting observation, which I

Table 8.9 **Menstrual regulation with vaginal administration of ONO-802**

Result:		
Treatment successful:	46 patients	
Treatment failed:	4 patients	
Total success rate:	92%	
No. of patients with positive pregnancy test before treatment;		31
No. of patients with successful treatment in this group:		27
Success rate:		87%
No. of patients with positive pregnancy test before treatment		19
No. of patients with successful treatment in this group:		19
Success rate:		100%

Source: reference 12

shall return to at the end of this presentation. When the data from the remaining 31 patients with confirmed pregnancy are examined, it can be seen that the success rate is actually 87%.

A much larger and more recent clinical trial of the use of Cervagem for menstrual regulation has recently been carried out in Indonesia[13]. A total of 534 patients were admitted, and the results are summarized in Table 8.10. We are fortunate to have with us today three of the investigators and they may wish to elaborate on their results during the discussion.

The results for menstrual regulation are, in general, very similar to

Table 8.10   Indonesian multicentre study

Patients admitted	534
Patients withdrawn	5
Menstrual-like bleeding induced	528/529
Patients requiring follow-up D & C	73/529
Failure of treatment	1/529

Source: reference 13

those obtained elsewhere in trials for termination of early pregnancy. The studies just described are being followed up in Indonesia by a much larger wide-scale clinical evaluation programme for Cervagem.

Additional evidence for the use of Cervagem in menstrual regulation has recently been obtained by our colleagues at the Ono Pharmaceutical Company in Japan, and I am indebted to them for allowing me to present their data. They have found that a 1 mg pessary of ONO-802 induces uterine contractions in non-pregnant women similar to those produced in pregnant women. This has led to an investigation of the ability of ONO-802 to induce menstrual bleeding at various times during the luteal phase in women[14]. The results obtained when ONO-802 was administered at various states of the menstrual cycle in nine women are shown in Table 8.11. Post-ovulatory doses were administered to the first three women in the early luteal phase of their menstrual cycle on days 1, 2 and 4 and, in these cases, no bleeding was observed, although two of the women reported the side-effects typical of

Table 8.11   Administration of ONO-802 vaginal suppository during the luteal phase of the menstrual cycle

Case no.	Length of usual menstrual cycle (days)	Day of dosing (day 0 = day of ovulation)	Dose	Time to onset of bleeding (hour/min)	Duration of bleeding (days)	Side-effects
1	30	1	1 mg × 5	—	—	Diarrhoea
2	30	2	1 mg × 5	—	—	—
3	28	4	1 mg × 5	—	—	Flushing
4	30	5	1 mg × 5	9° 20′	Spotting	Diarrhoea
5	28	6	1 mg × 5	—	—	—
6	30	9	1 mg × 4	10° 08′	Spotting	—
7	28	11	1 mg × 5	15° 21′	3	—
8	28	12	1 mg × 4	11° 43′	7	—
9	28	12	1 mg × 3	8° 25′	5	—

Source: reference 14

120

prostaglandins. Post-ovulatory dosing of three women on days 5, 6 and 9 (during the mid-luteal phase) produced spotting in two cases. When dosing was performed during the late luteal phase, on days 11 and 12 in the three cases studied, bleeding was induced in all three women, with an apparently normal duration of menstrual bleeding. The results suggest that ONO-802 can be used to interrupt the process of implantation of a fertilized ovum in the uterus. On day 14 post-ovulation, that is on the expected day of mestruation, the fertilized ovum is established in the endometrium, but it is not until day 21 post-ovulation that the chorionic villi are established. Thus, it is reasonable to postulate that administration of a menstrual regulator, such as Cervagem, 1 or 2 days after the expected day of menstruation, would lead to shedding of the endometrium together with the fertilized ovum into the menstrual blood flow. However, I must emphasize that much work still remains to be done to confirm this possibility.

During the next 12 months, we expect to obtain regulatory approval for ONO-802 in at least two indication in various countries around the world. Ome will be for pre-operative cervical dilatation in pregnant women. As I have mentioned, we are also continuing to test the efficacy of ONO-802 for cervical dilatation in non-pregnant women. The other approved indication we are seeking is for second trimester therapeutic termination of pregnancy. In addition, regulatory approval is expected by the Ono Pharmaceutical Co. for ONO-802 in Japan very soon for the indication of termination of second trimester pregnancy.

References

1 Sakamoto, S., Satoh, K., Nishiya, I., Kunimoto, K. *et al.* (1982). Abortifacient effect and uterine cervix-dilating action of 16,16-dimethyl-*trans*-Δ^2 PGE$_1$ methyl ester (ONO-802) in the form of a vaginal suppository (a randomised, double-blind, controlled study in the second trimester of pregnancy). *Prostaglandins Leukotrienes Med.*, **9**, 349.
2 Takagi, S., Yoshida, T., Ohya, A., Tsubata, K., Sakata, H., Fujii, K. T., Iizuka, S., Tochigi, B., Tochigi, M. and Mochigi, A. (1982). The abortifacient effect of 16,16-dimethyl-*trans*-Δ^2 PGE$_1$ methyl ester, a new prostaglandin analogue, on mid-trimester pregnancies and long-term follow-up observations. *Prostaglandins*, **23**, 591
3 Satoh, Y., Takahashi, T. and Takeuchi, S. (1981). Second trimester abortion by intravaginal administration of prostaglandin (ONO-802)*. *Gendai Iryo (Current Med.)*, **13**, 1215
4 Yamamoto, M., Sugimoto, T. and Kisohara, H. (1980). Experience of therapeutic termination of mid-trimester pregnancies by intravaginal administration of a prostaglandin E$_1$ analogue*. *Kanto District Branch J. Japan Obstet. Gynaecol. Soc.*, **32**, 38.
5 Hamada, T. and Taki, I. (1981). Expulsive effect of intravaginal administration of a prostaglandin E$_1$ analogue on second trimester uterine contents*. *Sanfujinka no Sekai (World of Obstet. Gynaecol.)*, **32**, 713

6 Migita, M., Hirakawa, O., Yakabe, A., Akita, S., Kuramoto, T., Nagaya, H., Torigoe, T. and Koresawa, M. (1980). Abortifacient effect of intravaginal administration of a prostaglandin E_1 analogue on second trimester pregnancies*. *Sanfujinka no Sekai (World of Obstet. Gynaecol.)*, **32**, 961

7 Affandi, B., Santoso, S. S. I., Moclock, F. A., Wibowo, B., Sumapraja, S. and Samil, R. S. (1981). Comparative study between saline instillation and vaginal pessary PG ONO-802 for second trimester abortion. Presented at the *8th Asian and Oceanic Congress of Obstetrics and Gynaecology*, October 25–31, Melbourne, Australia

8 Takagi, S., Sakata, H., Yoshida, T., Den, K., Fujii, T. K., Amemiya, H. and Tomita, M. (1978). Termination of early pregnancy by ONO-802 suppositories (16,16-dimethyl-*trans*-Δ^2 PGE_1 methyl ester). *Prostaglandins*, **15**, 913

9 Karim, S. M. M. (1979). Data on file at May & Baker Ltd., Dagenham, Essex, UK

10 The World Health Organization, Task Force on the Use of Prostaglandins for the Regulation of Fertility. Geneva, Switzerland (1982). Termination of early first trimester pregnancy by vaginal administration of 16,16-dimethyl-*trans*-Δ^2 PGE_1 methyl ester. *Asia-Oceania J. Obstet. Gynaecol.*, **8**, 263

11 Smith, S. K. and Baird, D. T. (1980). The use of 16,16-dimethyl-*trans*-Δ^2 PGE_1 methyl ester (ONO-802) vaginal suppositories for the termination of early pregnancy. A comparative study. *Br. J. Obstet. Gynaecol.*, **87**, 712

12 Karim, S. M. M., Ratnam, S. S. and Illancheran, A. (1977). Menstrual induction with vaginal administration of 16,16-dimethyl-*trans*-Δ^2 PGE_1 methyl ester (ONO-802). *Prostaglandins*, **14**, 615

13 Agoestina, T., Sastrawinata, A., Prayitno, W., Gouta, P. (1982). Menstrual regulation with prostaglandin (PG ONO-802) in Indonesia. (In preparation)

14 Ono Pharmaceutical Company (1977). Administration of ONO-802 vaginal suppositories during the luteal phase of the menstrual cycle. Data on file at May & Baker Ltd., Dagenham, Essex, UK

* In Japanese

Introduction:

Cervagem future development

A. SALEM

In this first Cervagem International Symposium we have heard today the detailed results of closely monitored, controlled clinical trials with this new product. In many cases it has been our good fortune to receive the information from the best possible source – the investigators themselves.

I should like to spend a few moments describing, briefly, May & Baker's proposal for the immediate future of Cervagem in South-east Asia. This plan seems to us to follow sensibly from the holding of today's symposium.

As practising doctors, you will be the first to appreciate, particularly with regard to your specialty, the events leading to and surrounding the birth of a new pharmaceutical preparation. I am referring essentially to the transition between its development and marketing. These two situations differ very greatly as to their implications to the clinician. The former involves the gathering of convincing evidence for the product's efficacy, reliability and safety, from carefully monitored phase III clinical trials which, in the case of Cervagem, have been conducted in several countries including Singapore and Hong Kong. In the marketing situation, patients will not generally be subjected to the same rigours of selection before treatment with the product, or surveillance after treatment. The position is such that we believe it is in the interest of patients, prescribing doctors and the product itself, if the first use of the product under normal prescribing conditions is monitored by the prescribing clinician. This can, of course, be kept within reasonable bounds and must be practicable to the busy doctor.

We trust that today's proceedings have provoked your interest, and it is our hope, during the course of the next few months, to be able to involve gynaecologists from this region in a large scale evaluation of Cervagem by the prescriber, under conditions of its application as they normally occur in your clinics. The object of this user evaluation is to obtain, from those who subscribe, simple but essential monitoring information on the behaviour of the product during normal prescribing use.

Our proposal covers two indications for Cervagem, namely, (a) preoperative cervical dilatation prior to surgical termination of pregnancy, and (b) therapeutic termination of second trimester pregnancy. It should, however, be noted in this context that legal, ethical or regulatory constraints which apply in different countries within South-east Asia will be respected and may govern the extent and timing of your individual participation.

We hope that the full benefit of this in-use evaluation can be derived by collection and publication of the results by the contributors to the study.

Mrs Susan Pitts, of May & Baker's Clinical Research Department, will now give a brief illustrated explanation of our recommendations for operating this programme for evaluation of Cervagem in clinical practice.

9
Cervagem future development: proposed clinical evaluation by the prescriber

S. A. PITTS

For the purpose of this evaluation, the normal prescribing information for Cervagem has been transcribed into a protocol format. Cervagem is indicated for *pre-operative cervical dilatation and second trimester therapeutic termination of pregnancy*, and the protocol is set out here.

PROTOCOL

Objectives	1. To evaluate cervical dilatation following administration of a single Cervagem 1mg pessary 3 to 4 hours pre-operatively. OR 2. To evaluate efficacy and side-effects of a course of 5 Cervagem 1mg pessaries over 12 hours for therapeutic termination of second trimester pregnancies.
	This drug must not be used for induction of labour at term.
1. Admissions	a. Women scheduled to undergo gynaecological operations which will require dilatation of cervix uteri. OR b. Women between 12 and 22 weeks pregnant who require therapeutic termination of pregnancy.
2. Exclusions	a. Patients with known sensitivity to prostaglandins. b. Pregnant patients in whom the pregnancy is expected to continue to term.
3. Precautions	Cervagem should be used with caution in patients with:- a. Obstructive airways disease. c. Elevated intraocular pressure. b. Cardiovascular insufficiency. d. Cervicitis or vaginitis.

Method
Examine and take history.

Cervical dilatation
a. Insert one Cervagem pessary into the posterior vaginal fornix 3-4 hours pre-operatively. Record time.
b. Record time of start of surgery.
c. Record size of largest dilator which can be inserted without force.
d. Assess further dilatation if needed as:
easy
average
difficult
e. Estimate blood loss.
f. Record operative procedure.
g. Record adverse reactions.
h. Record any additional therapy.

Second trimester termination of pregnancy
a. Insert one Cervagem pessary into the posterior vaginal fornix.
b. A further 1mg pessary should be inserted into the vagina 3 hourly until:
i. Products of conception are expelled, or
ii. A total of 5 pessaries have been given, or
iii. Unacceptable side-effects occur.
c. Assess abortion as:
complete, or
incomplete, or
failure.
d. Estimate blood loss.
e. Record adverse reactions.
f. Record any additional therapy.

Criteria for assessment for second trimester termination of pregnancy

Complete
Complete expulsion of the products of conception within 24 hours of administration of the first pessary OR partial expulsion not requiring further treatment.

Incomplete
Partial expulsion of the products of conception requiring further treatment.

Failure
Failure to expel any products of conception within 24 hours.
OR
adverse reactions of sufficient severity to warrant stopping treatment.

Treatment of failures: Normal hospital routine.

General

May & Baker will supply record cards and Cervagem 1mg vaginal pessaries.

Pessaries must be stored at less than 4°C. One pessary should be taken from the pack and the remainder returned to the refrigerator.

Completed record cards will be collected by a May & Baker representative.

Nothing in this protocol shall preclude the investigator from stopping treatment with Cervagem at any time.

However, as the embryopathic effects of Cervagem are not known, once a pessary has been administered to a pregnant woman, her pregnancy *must* be terminated.

PATIENT RECORD CARDS

Patient Record Cards have been designed for convenience in the completion of essential background, patient history and trial data, and are shown below.

Patient Record Card: preoperative cervical dilatation

Trial Centre	Investigator
Patient's Name	Date: Day ☐☐ Month ☐☐ Year ☐☐
Details of relevant medical history and physical condition. (See precautions section of Protocol)	Primigravid ☐ Multigravid ☐
	Date of last menstrual period
	Obstetric history and examination.
	Comments
	Time of pessary insertion:
	Time of start of operation:
DILATATION (check one)	SOUND ONLY ☐
	HEGAR No.
	OR PRATT No.
	OR No.
Was further dilatation necessary?	YES ☐ NO ☐ If yes, was it
	EASY ☐ AVERAGE ☐ DIFFICULT ☐
DETAILS OF OPERATION PERFORMED	
OPERATIVE BLOOD LOSS:	NONE ☐ LIGHT ☐ AVERAGE ☐ HEAVY ☐

Side-effects	Time	Medication

General Comments

Investigator's Signature

128

Patient Record Card: second trimester therapeutic termination of pregnancy

Trial Centre	Investigator
Patient's Name	Date: Day ☐☐ Month ☐☐ Year ☐☐

Details of relevant medical history and physical condition (See precautions section of Protocol)	Primigravid ☐ Multigravid ☐
	Weeks pregnant
	Obstetric history and examination.
	Comments (including pregnancy abnormalities e.g. foetal death).

Relevant pre-treatment test results (eg: Hb, WBC)

	Time given	Side-effects	Medication
1st Pessary			
2nd Pessary			
3rd Pessary			
4th Pessary			
5th Pessary			

EXPULSION _____ HOURS AFTER FIRST PESSARY

ESTIMATED BLOOD LOSS _____ ML.

Was the abortion   COMPLETE ☐   INCOMPLETE ☐   FAILURE ☐

TREATMENT OF INCOMPLETE AND FAILURE AND FINAL OUTCOME

FOLLOW-UP VISIT (RECORD ANY RELEVANT INFORMATION)

General Comments

Investigator's Signature

Further information available on request.
MAY & BAKER LTD.,
14 CHIN BEE ROAD, JURONG TOWN, PO BOX 21, SINGAPORE 9161. TEL: SINGAPORE 2656244

M&B May & Baker

*Cervagem is a trade mark of May & Baker Ltd Dagenham Essex England   P42E/1366

It must be stressed that the safety of gemeprost to the embryo or fetus has not yet been fully studied, and once the Cervagem pessary has been administered to a pregnant woman, her pregnancy must be terminated. Cervagem should not be used for induction of labour at term.

Discussion 4
and future developments

(23) **Dr Goh** (Malaysia): One of the clinical applications of PGs is to terminate molar pregnancy. I am wondering whether this is a safe method. This is a common problem here and the standard procedure really is to stimulate the uterus with oxytocin drip and at the same time perform a suction evacuation, whether the uterus is 20 weeks or even 30 weeks, and it strikes me as being rather dangerous to give these pessaries to cause contractions and patients start to bleed. As we have heard there is some evidence that it causes a lot of bleeding. Professor Karim is rather quiet on this issue. I was just wondering whether you could make a comment.

Dr Karim: Yes. The hospital where I work is divided into three units. The University Unit and one Government Unit have always used PGs for evacuating hydatidiform mole. The third Unit has chosen not to, they have considered it dangerous. Even in our three-country collaborative project, Singapore and Medan have used PGs for evacuating the mole without any problems. Kuala Lumpur for some reason, decided it wasn't safe and opted out of this study. I certainly agree with people who have said that one has to watch out for bleeding but I do not feel that the use of PGs is contraindicated.

Dr Crowshaw: We are hoping to build from our own experience with a specific PG that we mentioned – Cervagem – and from the amount of data that we have, we are encouraged but we would not be complacent about this. There will be careful monitoring of patients treated with Cervagem in order to assess more accurately the overall incidence of complications or success rates in these areas, so it will be watched very carefully in the future as well.

Dr Fylling: I refer to a history of this particular WHO study some years ago when the first patient was a colleague and she had an extra-uterine pregnancy. At least in Scandinavia, the incidence of tubal pregnancy is increasing. I feel that if we use PGs in this case of early pregnancy, we will end up in some trouble sometimes with an early tubal pregnancy.

Dr Bygdeman: I agree that if you terminate early pregnancy there is a risk that there could be an extra-uterine pregnancy, but I think that is the same if you use vacuum aspiration or if you use PGs. You can't evacuate extra-uterine pregnancy by vacuum either. There is no difference between the two methods.

Dr Karim: We have had two cases of extra-uterine pregnancies. One of these was treated with Cervagem. According to the protocol for this particular study, the patient came to the hospital and one vaginal pessary was administered in the hospital by the doctor and she was given four to use herself. The patient came back the same evening, not having used any more pessaries, with bleeding, excruciating pain. The doctor on duty suspected extra-uterine pregnancy. The second one I can't remember the details, but nothing disastrous happened, but I certainly take your point that this is something that is going to be missed. We do know that most PGs that stimulate the uterus will also stimulate the tubes and may initiate bleeding and pain.

Dr Crowshaw: Would any one like to comment on the use of prostaglandins for dilating a non-pregnant cervix?

Dr Chow (Malaysia): I have experience with two cases with primary infertility. They came with a history of having had an attempt by a previous colleague who had to do a tubal insufflation on them and had failed to dilate the cervix. I used a PGE_2 tablet as a premedication and I succeeded in dilating the cervix. It is difficult for me to really come to a scientific conclusion that the PGE$_2$ had been fully responsible for the success I had in dilating the cervix. It could be that the previous gynaecologist's attempt at dilating the cervix made subsequent dilatation easy. Based on this experience, I think I would use PG if ever I am faced with the same problem again.

Dr Karim: I recollect that some years ago Dr Sivasamboo did some work in ten patients for dilating the cervix and the results were positive.

Chairman's concluding remarks

I am sure all of you will agree with me that this has been a stimulating afternoon. I am not going to detain you any longer by summarizing this afternoon's proceedings which will be published later.

On behalf of all the participants I would like to thank May & Baker Ltd for organizing the symposium, thank the speakers, particularly those from overseas, for their presentation, to those who took part in the discussion and to you all for attending the symposium. May I suggest we adjourn to the lounge and carry on with the discussion there, informally.

Sultan M. M. Karim

10
Preoperative cervical dilatation by vaginal pessaries containing a prostaglandin E₁ analogue (gemeprost, Cervagem)

M. G. ELDER

INTRODUCTION

Surgical termination of pregnancy by cervical dilatation and suction during the first trimester is a commonly performed operation. The incidence of subsequent mid-trimester abortions due to cervical damage at the time of cervical dilatation has been shown to increase[1], particularly in nulliparous patients[2]. A fast-acting locally administered non-invasive agent, used pre-operatively, which could soften and dilate the cervix should reduce the incidence of cervical damage which, in nulliparous patients, can be as high as 2.7%[3]. Prostaglandins have been shown to lower the resistance of the cervix to mechanical dilatation[4], and to reduce the stretch modulus of human cervical tissue *in vitro*[5]. The mechanism of action may be due to alterations in the composition of collagen ground substance[6]. Prostaglandin E_2 has been used in this role but large doses are required which cause troublesome side-effects[7]. The intravaginal administration of a potent prostaglandin analogue may be efficacious with an acceptably low incidence of side-effects. This paper reports two studies of the use of a single intravaginal pessary of 16,16-dimethyl-*trans*-Δ^2 PGE_1 methyl ester (gemeprost) inserted approximately 3 hours before surgical termination of first trimester pregnancies.

PATIENTS AND METHODS

Two studies have been carried out: the first involved 43 patients who were pregnant for the first time and who had not had any operations involving the cervix. All were between 7 and 12 weeks pregnant as assessed by the period of amenorrhoea and by clinical assessment of uterine size. The study was an open one comparing the effects of a single Cervagem intravaginal pessary containing 1 mg gemeprost inserted 3 hours pre-operatively with a control group of patients who received no treatment prior to surgery. There were 25 patients in the study group and 18 patients in the control group, allocation being on a random basis. The second study was a double-blind placebo-controlled study involving 108 patients of whom 39 were primigravidae and 69 multigravidae. All were between 7 and 13 weeks pregnant as assessed by the period of amenorrhoea and by clinical assessment of uterine size. Either one pessary containing 1 mg gemeprost or a matching placebo pessary was inserted approximately 3 hours pre-operatively.

The force in kilograms needed to insert each cervical dilator fully was measured by means of a spring gauge attached to its handle. Pressure between the operator's hand, principally the thenar eminence, and the butt of the spring gauge caused compression of the spring, the force being registered directly on a scale from 0.3–1.2 kg by a pointer which did not return when the force ceased to be applied. To minimize error only two surgeons were involved in each study. Once adequate cervical dilatation had been obtained the pregnancy was terminated by vacuum aspiration. Operative blood loss was measured. The statistical significant of the difference of the results between the two groups was assessed by Student's t test or Mann–Whitney U test as appropriate.

RESULTS

Study 1

There were no significant differences between the treatment and control groups in mean age, gestation at time of termination of pregnancy, clinical assessment of uterine size, and blood loss at operation (Table 10.1). The reduction in the cervical resistance to the passage of a dilator was assessed by determining the maximum diameter of dilator that could be passed with a force of less than 0.3 kg, the smallest recordable force registered on the spring gauge. The force required to

Table 10.1 Age, gestation, uterine size and operative blood loss for treatment and control groups

	Treatment group (n = 25)	Control group (n = 18)	
Age	20.6 ± 4.4	21.9 ± 4.6	n.s.
Gestation (days)	75.9 ± 11.7	71.5 ± 9.7	n.s.
Clinically assessed uterine size	10.1 ± 1.2	9.9 ± 1.5	n.s.
Operative blood loss (ml)	130.4 ± 100.4	108.9 ± 43.0	n.s.

Values are mean ± 1 SD
n.s. = no significant difference between mean values

Table 10.2 Dilatation of the cervix in treatment and control groups

	Treatment group (n = 25)	Control group (n = 18)	Statistical significance of difference between groups
Maximum diameter of dilator inserted with no recordable pressure (mm)	6.4 ± 2.8	4.1 ± 2.4	$p < 0.001$
Force required to insert maximum size of dilator (kg)	0.9 ± 0.3	1.2 ± 0.2	$p < 0.001$

Values are mean ± 1 SD

insert the maximum size of dilator needed was recorded for both treatment and control groups (Table 10.2). Pre-operative side-effects in the form of mild or moderate preoperative pain and bleeding were experienced by 44% of the treatment group. Only 12% of patients were nauseated and 4% vomited. No symptoms were reported preoperatively in the control group.

Study 2

There were no significant differences between the treatment and control group in terms of age, parity and gestation. Operative time and bleeding was significantly reduced in the treatment group compared with controls (Table 10.3). The maximum diameter of dilator that could be passed with a force of less than 0.3 kg being registered on the spring gauge and the force required to insert the maximum size of

Table 10.3 Age, parity, gestation and uterine size for treatment and control groups

	Treatment group (n = 54)	Control group (n = 54)	
Age	24.5 ± 6.6 (range: 15–39)	25.1 ± 5.7 (range: 14–38)	n.s.
Parity	1.0 ± 1.3 (range: 0–6)	1.2 ± 1.3 (range: 0–5)	n.s.
Gestation (weeks)	10.1 ± 1.5	10.5 ± 1.7	n.s.
Operation time (min)	7.6 ± 2.2	9.4 ± 2.8	$p < 0.001$
Operative bleeding (ml)	118.1 + 51.8	196.1 ± 121.3	$p < 0.001$

Values are mean ± 1 SD
n.s. = no significant difference between the two groups

Table 10.4 Dilatation of the cervix in treatment and control groups

	Treatment group (n = 54)	Control group (n = 54)	Statistical significance of difference between groups
Maximum diameter of dilator inserted with no recordable pressure (mm)	8.9 ± 2.6	6.6 ± 1.7	$p < 0.001$
Number of dilators necessary for further dilatation	2.4 ± 2.2	4.5 ± 1.7	$p < 0.001$
Force required to insert maximum size of dilator (kg)	0.73 ± 0.54	1.13 ± 0.21	$p < 0.001$

Values are mean ± 1 SD

dilator needed are shown in Table 10.4. In the treatment group 47% of patients experienced mild abdominal pain and slight bleeding pre-operatively. Four per cent of patients in the treatment group vomited.

DISCUSSION

Mechanical dilatation of the cervix, particularly in nulliparous patients, can be difficult and in a few cases will lead to obvious cervical lacerations, but in a substantial number of others cervical damage may be unnoticed and cause subsequent mid-trimester abortions and preterm labour. This study has shown clearly that the pre-operative use of a vaginal pessary of PGE_1 analogue causes significant softening and dilatation of the cervix in most patients, allowing for the insertion without resistance of, on average, a 6 mm diameter dilator in nulliparous patients and 9 mm in a group of patients of mixed parity. Mild pain and bleeding is initiated by the prostaglandin analogue but this is not troublesome. The incidence of gastro-intestinal side-effects is insignificant. The pessary should be left *in situ* for at least 3 hours to allow for maximum dilatation.

References

1 Richardson, J. A., and Dixon, G. (1976). Effects of legal termination on subsequent pregnancy. *Br. Med. J.,* **1**, 1303
2 Harlap, S., Shiono, P. H., Ramcharan, S. *et al.* (1979). A prospective study of spontaneous fetal loss after induced abortions. *N. Engl. J. Med.,* **301**, 677
3 Atienza, M. F., Burkman, R. T., and King, T. M. (1980). Forces associated with cervical dilatation at suction abortion. Qualitative and quantitative data in studies completed with a force sensing instrument. In Naftolin, F. and Stubblefield, P. D. (eds.) *Dilatation of the Uterine Cervix*, pp. 343–354. New York: Raven Press
4 Dingfelder, J. R., Brenner, W. E., Hendricks, C. H. and Stavrovsky, L. G. (1975). Reduction of cervical resistance by prostaglandin suppositories prior to dilatation for induced abortion. *Am. J. Obstet. Gynecol.,* **122**, 25
5 Conrad, J. T. and Euland, K. (1976). Reduction of the stretch modulus of human cervical tissue by prostaglandin E_2. *Am. J. Obstet. Gynecol.,* **126**, 218
6 Danforth, D. N., Veis, A., Breen, M. *et al.* (1974). The effect of pregnancy and labour on the human cervix: Changes in collagen, glycoproteins and glycosamino glycans. *Am. J. Obstet. Gynecol.,* **120**, 641
7 MacKenzie, I. Z. and Fry, A. (1981). Prostaglandin E_2 pessaries to facilitate first trimester aspiration termination. *Br. J. Obstet. Gynaecol.,* **88**, 1033

Index